The Influence of Christians in Medicine

THE INFLUENCE OF CHRISTIANS IN MEDICINE

Edited by
J. T. Aitken, H. W. C. Fuller and D. Johnson

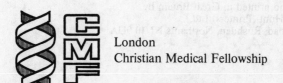

London
Christian Medical Fellowship

© Christian Medical Fellowship

First published 1984

Christian Medical Fellowship
157 Waterloo Road, London SE1 8XN

ISBN 0 906747 11 2

Trade Agents:
INTER-VARSITY PRESS
Norton Street
Nottingham NG7 3HR

Photoset and printed in Great Britain by
Stanley L. Hunt (Printers) Ltd.
Midland Road, Rushden, Northants NN10 9UA

C. GORDON SCORER

M.B.E., M.D., F.R.C.S. (Edin. & Eng.)

THIS book is a tribute to the memory of Charles Gordon Scorer, known affectionately to colleagues and countless friends across the world for his wise counsel and meticulously careful writing on matters surgical and spiritual. He was one of the chief of those involved in the planning of the triad of books: *Decision Making in Medicine, The Influence of Christians in Medicine* and *The Bible and Medicine,* of which this is the second to appear. The authors hope that all these volumes will reflect his conviction that the Bible is our surest guide in matters of faith and conduct.

PREFACE

THE thesis of this book is that Western Medicine, from the fourth century A.D. to the present day, has owed a great debt to Christianity and to individual Christians for the maintenance of its tradition and progress. While fully recognizing the early and parallel debts to Greek, Jewish and Arabic Medicine, the writers have brought together historical evidence for their claim. The material is extensive and the chief difficulty has been one of selection.

One aspect of this problem has been the need accurately to define the word Christian both in reference to an individual practitioner and the social community in which he worked. A similar problem presented itself in seeking to assess the general state and spiritual health of the Christian religious communities at any one time. Clues for these have been sought in the more scanty sources available for details of the family background and denominational affiliation of those included. Biographical materials for these are comparatively scarce for the first 1500 years of the Christian era. Even in recent times the standard biographies often show considerable reticence in mentioning the subject of religion. The writers have, therefore, taken the view that in the earlier years of Church history the word Christian must be taken in a more formal and general sense. But in the later chapters they have looked more closely for evidence of Church attendance and personal Christian commitment in their exemplars. The general aim throughout has been to include those who have clearly come under the influence of the life and teachings of Christ.

Two important aspects in medical and Christian history have been intentionally omitted. One of these is the Church and faith healing. The reason for excluding this is that we are concerned here with the influence of Christians in orthodox Medicine. The place of the supernatural in relation to the day-to-day decisions and procedures of an individual practitioner or hospital has been voluminously discussed elsewhere. The subject is more within the ambit of Church history than that of Medicine.

The second omission is of any reference to the later progress of psychological medicine. The Church and its representatives have exercised an extensive and beneficent role not only in support of those needing psychiatric care, but in the maintenance of the spiritual factor in the experience of those concerned. In the student and adolescent world writings such as those of Gordon W. Allport, Professor of Psychology at Harvard University (see his *The Individual and His Religion*) have proved of suggestive value in this direction. There have been others who have sought to come to terms with the basic problems of relating spirit and mind from the Christian point of view. The subject demands much greater space than could be given here.

Acknowledgements

It is impossible to do justice to the help received from all who have contributed suggestions, responded to enquiries concerning historical detail and assisted in other ways. Some, however, have gone to extra trouble in their correspondence and must be cited. It should be made clear that none of these is responsible for the form in which their material has been included or for opinions expressed.

The Editors wish especially to thank the following overseas correspondents, Dr. R. Bastian (Deutsches Institut für Arztliche Mission, Tübingen); Professor John Brobeck (Philadelphia); Miss Marguerite Bronkema (Librarian, Missionary Study Center, Ventnor, N.J.); Dr. Ernst Harnick (Zürich); Professor R. Hooykaas (Zeist); Professor Hilmar Iversen (Oslo); Mr. Paul Jenkins (Basler Mission); Professor G. A. Lindeboom (Amsterdam); Dr. Eleonore Lippits (Aachen); Dr. Børg Marner (Copenhagen); Dr. Karl L. Mettinger (Stockholm); Dr. C. Tucker (Wellington, N.Z.); and, also, in the British Isles Dr. Roy Billington (London); Dr. James Broomhall (Crowborough, Sussex); the late Dr. Frank Davey (the Methodist Missionary Society); Dr. Helen Eaton (Glasgow); Lt. Col. S. L. Gauntlet (Salvation Army); Mr. J. T. Handyman (British Council of Churches, London); Mr. Douglas Jackson (Birmingham); Professor Ian Porter (Aberdeen); Sr. Maria Teresa Reilly (Medical Missionaries of Mary, Dundalk); Dr. Colin Russell (the Open University); Dr. David S. Short (Aberdeen); and Miss F. H. B. Williams (the Selly Oak Colleges' Library). Tribute is also due to the patient and cheerful members of the library staffs at the Royal College of Physicians, the Royal College of Surgeons, the Royal Society of Medicine and the Wellcome Institute of the History of Medicine. Not least, special thanks are due to the Rev. John Rivers (Cley, Norfolk) who made ready for the press and Miss Marjorie Watling (Sutton, Surrey), who typed and retyped the manuscript.

THE EDITORS.

CONTENTS

CONTENTS

CHAPTER 1

CHRISTIANITY AND MEDICINE :
NATURAL ALLIES

ALL essential occupations offer, in different forms, true service to mankind. At first sight, however, some appear more obviously to be in keeping with the spirit and practice of the Christian faith. Among these, apart from the ordained Christian ministry, Medicine has tended to take pride of place. For in several ways doctors and nurses have an especially close rapport with those whom they serve, and Christians in both these professions have unique opportunities to express the ideals inspired by their faith. This circumstance has no doubt been one of the chief underlying factors which has encouraged so many Christians down the centuries to offer their services to humanity in the ranks of Medicine and Nursing. Historical records make clear that during the development of Western civilization the Christian Church played a considerable part in the progress of patient care and the advances of scientific Medicine.

FORMS OF SERVICE

There are other beneficent ways in which Christians have made worthy contributions, besides the sheer weight of the numbers serving. One of them is finance. During the early centuries of the Christian era, and again in the 18th and 19th centuries (when the State was making very meagre, if any, provision for the sick poor), it was the Church which made possible the building of large numbers of 'hospices' and 'hospitals'. Voluntary collections for the poor, the sick, and hospitals were regularly taken at the Sunday services and during some of the Church's festivals. And, when free hospitals were built, it was, at least initially, a Christian impulse which encouraged the physicians and surgeons to give their services freely. From such beginnings developed the great Voluntary Hospitals of the 19th century.

Another way in which the Faith has deeply influenced day to day practice of Medicine is through its power to motivate for corporate service to the community as well as to the individual. The teachings of Christ and his apostles are explicit in their emphasis upon a Christian's duty to love his neighbour. Hence it is not surprising to find that, in those periods when the spiritual health of the Church has been at its best, its practical influence in the medical world has been correspondingly evident. This was convincingly shown during the 19th and early part of the 20th centuries by the response of the Christians in Europe and North America to the medical needs of the developing countries of the Third World.

It is not only in the form of such practical actions that the effects have been seen, but also in the more theoretical spheres of the regulation of professional procedures and conduct. For, while the Hippocratic Oath (bequeathed from the golden age of Greek Medicine) has been traditionally and widely acknowledged and, in a few universities, required by the official medical authorities to be sworn by those newly qualified, growth in ethical standards has been slow. In the experience of many individual practitioners it has been the influence of general Christian ethics which has quietly and soundly guided them in their daily work. For what could be more relevant than the basic principle stated by Christ in Mark 12.29-31 (and more briefly as the Golden Rule in Matthew 7.12) — 'In everything do to others what you would have them do to you, for this sums up the Law and the Prophets.'

INTELLECTUAL STIMULUS

There have been other ways in which, directly and indirectly, Christianity has influenced Medicine, only one of which need be mentioned here. A search into the early life and education of many of the prominent pioneers in modern Medicine reveals a number of interesting and significant facts. Some of the more virile and farsighted among them experienced strong religious influence from their families or in university days. Contrary to popular opinion today, this factor proved itself to be a strong intellectual stimulus to their scientific curiosity, originality and industry in research. Such a possibility is strikingly argued in a book published recently as a tribute to the late George Rosen, the distinguished Jewish medical historian. The chapter by E. H. Ackerknecht of Zürich entitled *German Jews, English Dissenters, French Protestants: Nineteenth Century Pioneers of Modern Medicine and Science* lists the many successful men of scientific genius produced by these distinctive communities and asks what influences, shared by these minorities, may have been most responsible for the quite outstanding contributions which they have made. Professor

Ackerknecht attributes it to the religious persecution and other adverse circumstances which each minority suffered, and especially to the severe social discrimination which they had to overcome. Among these were laws excluding them from the universities or from holding posts in any of them, or indeed from holding any government post.

We would ask, however, whether this was so clearly the cause or the only cause. For elsewhere in the world and among other religious minorities similar pressures have not necessarily produced comparable effects. While they are not exact parallels, there have been many persecuted minority religions in Asia (especially the Indian subcontinent) and Africa where comparable effects have not been seen. But there is one exception which would seem significant in this context: members of the Coptic Church in Egypt, in spite of many pressures, have achieved high standards in Science and Medicine.

There is another common factor which is shared by these Jewish and Christian minorities. Each of them has been deeply influenced by the Bible, though this for the Jews means solely the Old Testament. Each group was educated in a strong biblical Theism, that is in a firm belief in a personal God who is the sovereign Creator of the universe and of man. From evidence in the biographies of many men of genius, Theism has proved a powerful incentive to scholarly and scientific activity. Since God has encouraged man to look into his creation, the Christian and Jewish Theist has a fertile incentive to do so. Their research is pursued within a theological and philosophical framework which accepts the evidence for design and a providential maintenance of the universe. Hence they work in an orderly world not subject to the caprice of pagan deities or mere chance. The Bible also supplies a stimulus for the Theist's application to basic research. In general it also impresses on the devout mind the ethical duty of altruistic service in applying the results of their research to the well-being of neighbours and the community. It is, therefore, apparent that the Bible through its teaching concerning the sovereign Creator embodies a principle which has been of vital importance in much modern scientific and medical discovery, and which deserves re-assessment in the light of the evidence. Both Jews and Christians have made many major contributions to the charitable care of sick persons. They have been, and are still, found at the growing points in Medicine.

OUR AIM

In what follows it is not intended to trace again the central story of

Medicine, for this has been done, and well done, by a number of medical historians fully equipped for the task. The purpose of this book is to describe some of the more important points at which Christian influence or individual Christians have been responsible for advances in patient care or scientific treatment. With its distinctive outlook Christianity has been the natural ally of Medicine and it has been active on a world scale.

The field of Medicine is in itself international and transcends differing cultures and classes. Various schools of thought of many backgrounds have made their contributions to the irregular and unequal steps by which Medicine has advanced into modern times. As Oliver Wendell Holmes writes, 'The truth is that Medicine, professedly founded on observation, is as sensitive to outside influences — political, religious, philosophical and imaginative — as is the barometer to the changes in atmospheric density. Theoretically it ought to go on its own straightforward inductive path without regard to changes of government or fluctuations in public opinion . . . (yet there is) a closer relation between the Medical Sciences and the conditions of society and the general thought of the time than would at first be suspected.'

We have, therefore, to look behind the records of the personalities concerned to their origins and the circumstances of their day to make any valid assessment of the sources of their inspiration. William Osler, a former Regius Professor of Medicine at Oxford, commented: 'It is only by the historical method that many of the intellectual problems in Medicine can be approached.' It will, therefore, be necessary in what follows to note the general movement of scientific Medicine in the Christian era from the Greek and Roman cities to Alexandria and the Arabic world of the Near East and back to the cities of Western Europe and, later, America.

The search has repeatedly confirmed in the minds of the writers the conviction that the apparent affinity between Christianity and Medicine is not simply a matter of superficial appearance. What has proved to be such a fruitful co-operation is more than the fortuitous results of a working partnership. In principle the ideals for sound scientific Medicine and the best clinical care are very similar to those which, in the spiritual realm, hold for the Christian faith, which has proved itself such a unique source of motivation for service to humanity.

THE IMPORTANCE OF HISTORY

In 1769, at a time when medical practice had once again begun to show signs of advance, the London physician John Fothergill wrote to a fellow member of the Religious Society of Friends: 'Let us preserve the memory of the deserving, perhaps it may prompt others to deserve.' This comment is salutary, for public memory is short and human nature needs repeated stimulus. Something of what is needed has been best preserved in some of Medicine's art treasures.

In many homes at the beginning of the century was a copy of Sir Luke Fildes' poignant painting known as *The Doctor,* now in the Tate Gallery. In the shade of the lamp a pensive family practitioner is watching a seriously ill child at the crisis of a fever. In the background are the shadows of the distressed parents awaiting the verdict. In more recent times their anxiety might well have been less. For even then rapid advances were already taking place towards higher degrees of specialization in most branches of Medicine and the highly skilled specialist was ready to supplement the work of the general practitioner. Hence, early in the 20th century, it was more appropriate to display in the hall of the Welch Memorial Library of the Johns Hopkins Hospital, Baltimore, the well known painting of *The Four Doctors,* or *The Big Four.* Each pioneered advances in his own department when the 'Hopkins' was at the crest of its fame: William Osler (medicine), William S. Halsted (surgery), Howard A. Kelly (gynaecology) and William H. Welch (pathology).

Since that time interest has become focused more on the highly trained teams which are involved in today's specialist diagnoses and treatments. Something of this modern team concept has been caught in the stained glass window which impresses a visitor entering the hall of the Foundation Building at the Mayo Clinic, Rochester, Minnesota. Panels side by side illustrate the three main lines of advance in the fields of medical education, medical practice and medical research. The central panel bears the inscription — 'To cure sometimes, to relieve often, to comfort always'. Over the centuries many Christians have been at the growing points, helping to increase the numbers relieved and, if possible, cured. The task, however, is far from finished. Let us trust that the future will see increasingly fruitful initiatives by devout Christians in the care of sick persons throughout the world.

CHAPTER 2

HOSPITAL FOUNDING AND FUNDING

OF all the ways in which Christians have, on a world scale, served the interests of medical care, none is more obvious than their industry in building hospitals. From the fourth century A.D. until the 20th century this activity has been a constant feature of their concern and there have been prolonged periods when such hospital-building movements have added significantly to existing provisions for the sick and underprivileged. From small beginnings the process reached epidemic proportions in the 19th century. It was not simply a matter of planning and siting the new institutions, but also involved the more difficult task of raising sufficient funds for the cost of their building and maintenance. History throws into relief five main periods in which work was done, but before considering them, and in order to retain due perspective, two explanations are necessary.

The first dates for which we are able to trace Christian hospital foundations come in the fourth century A.D. This may seem unduly late, and prompts the question — why were Christians so long in showing evidence of the philanthropic virtues claimed for them? The reasons were political and social. For until the Emperor Constantine had granted the first Edict of Toleration in A.D. 311 (further extended by later legislation in 313) they were subject to discrimination which permitted little room for manoeuvre and left them with small economic resources. From time to time, depending on the Emperor's outlook and character, there was the fiercest official persecution which brought the death penalty for refusal to worship the Emperor as god. Only when toleration was finally granted could political freedom and access to adequate resources allow the Christians to express themselves freely and to develop their own typical institutions.

Then, in the optimistic and expansionist outlook of the 19th century it was commonly claimed that it was the early Christians who built the first hospitals. However the 'hospices' (guest houses for the sick and chronically disabled) in primitive times were different from the modern hospital, and active successful treatments were few. History suggests, in fact, that the 'hospital' antedated the Christian era.

CHRISTIANITY'S PREDECESSORS

It is claimed that 'hospitals' in the East were built by Buddhists as far back as the year 260 B.C. and that several were founded by the Emperor Asoka in Hindustan before 232 B.C. Similarly, 'hospitals' of some kind existed in regions where Brahministic medicine was practised early in antiquity, and two in Sri Lanka have been dated as early as 431 B.C. and 137 B.C. respectively. From classical sources it also seems that, many years before Christ, there were in the Near East 'hospitals' attached to the temples of Saturn. Their reputation drew large numbers of sufferers to the more popular centres such as Heliopolis, Memphis and Thebes. These centres, of course, would primarily have offered accommodation for sleep in the temple precincts and a visit would have been more like a modern pilgrimage to the shrine at Lourdes. During the main period of Greek civilization a proto-hospital developed at the temple of Asklepios at Cos. There were similar institutions at Cnidos, Epidaurus, Athens, Rhodes and Pergamon.

In Rome a temple of healing was erected on an island in the Tiber, later to be called St. Bartholomew's because of the Christian church that was eventually built there. At subsequent stages in the history of the Empire, military hospitals (*valetudinaria*) for the Roman legions were to be found in most of the chief garrison towns. There are also incidental comments in the descriptions of later Rome which might suggest that some *valetudinaria* had also been established in the major cities for the treatment of civilians. During the excavations of the ruins of Pompeii (destroyed in A.D. 79) a doctor's house was found, which seems to have been like a small nursing home.

THE ESSENTIAL CHRISTIAN CONTRIBUTION

The typical attitude to the sick on the part of the early Christians was based on Christ's parable of the Good Samaritan. It highlights the place of mercy or compassion in relation to any neighbour in need. It stands for all time as a lesson for all nations and not only for Jews and Christians. There is some evidence that even before the grant of their new liberties in the fourth century the Christians had begun to change for the better the prevailing attitude to the sick, disabled and handicapped. There are also indications that in cities where Christians were at all numerous they had begun to set up 'hospices' for the chronically ill, and that a few of these were already being designated as hospices reserved for sufferers from 'leprosy'. This is a disease which has received particular interest from the Church throughout the centuries, from the example set by Christ.

By the time of Tertullian the various charitable outlets for Christian love, to which the congregations were exhorted to commit themselves, had become quite extensive. Even the pagans could comment 'How these Christians love one another'. As Tertullian explains: 'Every man once a month brings some modest coin, or whenever he wishes and only if he does wish, and if he can — for nobody is compelled.' He continues that the resulting funds were spent 'not on banquets and drinking parties' but 'to feed the poor and bury them, for boys and girls who have no resources or parents, for slaves who have grown old and shipwrecked sailors; and any who may be in the mines, on the islands in penal servitude, in prison, . . . they become the pensioners of their confession'.

In discussing the appeal of the new religion to ordinary members of the public amid the social tensions of a declining empire, H. E. Sigerist, the eminent Jewish medical historian, writes: 'The very fact that there was such an immense proletariat in the Roman Empire created a most fertile ground for the acceptance and spread of Christianity, a religion which addressed itself not only to the pure, but also to the underdog and promised healing, redemption, and equality before God.' The result was that: 'The most important and decisive development in the special status assigned to the sick was introduced by Christianity. This new teaching, in contrast with the other religions for the healthy and just man, appealed to the sick, to the weak and to the crippled. It spoke of spiritual healing, but it also spoke of bodily healing.'

Sigerist emphasizes that this Christian outlook brought a new dynamic force to society which held the promise of much future good. He writes: 'The place of the sick in society was altered from its very foundation. Whereas disease in the entire course of previous historical development had sharply isolated the sufferer, in Christian times he was actually brought closer to his fellow men by the fact of his illness. The diseased person is a man who has become a participant of the grace of God. To care for him is a Christian obligation, is positively beneficial to the salvation of his soul. The birth-hour of large-scale, organized care of the sick had come. The care of the ill is now the concern of the church. The bishop is in charge; the deacons and widows are his active agents. On Sundays, free-will offerings are collected for the sick and the poor of the church community. From the fourth century on, hospitals were constructed which were not founded on economic considerations, as had been the Roman slave and military hospitals. They were, on the contrary, to prove a clear expression of Christian charity.'

PERIODS OF HOSPITAL BUILDING

Over the centuries there have been times when Christian involvement in building activity has been more pronounced than at others. There have also been considerable differences between the types of central institution which have been produced. Much has depended on the aims of the founders, the circumstances of the times and the economic resources of those contributing to the cost. The periods of activity can be roughly classified into five main groups as follows: (1) early initiatives, 313-476 (that is, from the Edicts of Constantine until the fall of Rome); (2) the Dark Ages (476-1000); (3) the medieval hospitals (1000-1500); (4) from the 16th to 18th centuries (1500-1800), and (5) the 19th and 20th centuries (1800-the present).

It will make for greater clarity when we come to discuss the various institutions if the derivation of certain related terms can be observed. The words 'hospice', 'hotel' and 'hospital' each come originally from the same root, represented by the Latin *hospes* (a guest). A 'hospice' was a place for guests, such as, for example, the buildings attached to monasteries for use by the pilgrims. Through late French it developed into the familiar 'hotel' for 'guests' who paid an economic charge. It was probably from *hospitium* (hospitality) that came the words 'spital' and 'hospital', that is, a place for guests who were chronically sick or disabled. The latter in its original form is believed to have been an extra building to the monks' 'infirmary', supplying a hall for the pilgrims or other guests who might become ill, so that they could be attended by the lay monks who professed medicine as their vocation.

PERIOD 1: THE EARLIEST INITIATIVES (313-476)

St. Basil of Caesarea (in Cappadocia) deserves to be regarded as the pioneer in the first large-scale Christian movement for the care of the seriously ill and disabled. F. H. Garrison writes: 'In A.D. 369 the celebrated Basilica at Caesarea (Cappadocia) was founded by St. Basil, consisting of a large number of buildings, with houses for physicians and nurses, workshops and industrial schools. It was followed by a charity hospital of 300 beds for the plague stricken at Edessa, which was founded by St. Ephraim in 375.' St. Basil's hospital at Caesarea was a considerable concentration of buildings. For it included hospices for travellers, a hospice for the poor, a hospice for the aged, an isolation unit and a house for those suffering from leprosy, who were treated in isolation. As a result of St. Basil's advocacy, hospitals were also built in many Near-eastern cities. Sometimes, in the Eastern part of the Empire, this was with the assistance of the state.

This period of momentum in the founding of Christian hospitals came none too soon, for in 335 Constantine had issued a decree calling for the closure of all the hospital-type shrines dedicated to Asklepios which were attached to the pagan temples and popularly used for temple medicine. Had they not been replaced by the new Christian hospitals, many sick folk would have been left with no place of refuge. It is interesting to note that Constantine's own mother, Helena, is reputed to have been prominent among those who were helping to provide Christian aid. With the gifts of the richer Christians the Church was now able to establish a series of new-style *valetudinaria* for the public. Just as in Basil's institution there was often a group of buildings around some of these larger 'hospitals', which included houses for orphans and those of advanced age.

In the following century a series of monastery-based hospitals, often also accompanied by buildings for orphans and for the elderly, sprang up in many new cities. The first in Western Europe is believed to have been one in Rome founded by Fabriola about the year A.D. 400. She is said herself to have become one of its nurses. St. Jerome commented that she aimed 'to gather in the sick from the streets and to nurse the wretched sufferers, wasted with poverty and disease'. It is also noteworthy that the Empress Eudoxia is recorded as having been responsible for setting up a similar Christian hospital in Jerusalem. This ambitious hospital movement continued steadily for a number of years until its activities were halted by the depredations of the barbarian invaders, and the contemporary political and economic disasters of the Empire.

PERIOD 2: MONASTIC HOSPITALS OF THE DARK AGES (476-1000)

The 500 years following the fall of Rome in 476, commonly known as the Dark Ages, were not all gloom. Chiefly as a result of Christian influences three of the rulers took a lead in the right direction so far as medicine was concerned. Childebert, son of the King of the Franks, founded the Hôtel

Dieu in Lyons, while Theodoric the Great farsightedly sought to rebuild in his empire as many of the Roman type hospitals (*nosocomia*) as could be revived. He also encouraged any Christian initiatives concerned to set up hospitals. Charlemagne, however, proved the most enlightened of them all. He promulgated a decree that a school, monastery and hospital should be built, attached to every cathedral throughout his dominions. The extent to which this measure was put fully into practice is not clear, but some of the cities are certainly known to have had hospitals attached to the cathedral monasteries.

It was in 529 that a further major step in hospital-building and its organization was taken. St. Benedict of Nursia founded a monastery at Monte Cassino in Southern Italy, with a hospital attached. He made it clear from the start that the duty of his monks was to give primary attention to serving the seriously ill, and his rule was that 'the care of the sick is to be attended to before all things'. His rule was destined to become the model for many other later monastic establishments. In later times the Benedictine Order was principally to specialize in the care of the sick. The Benedictine pattern was adopted by their successors in the monastic tradition and expressed in the following terms: '*Care for the sick stands before and over all*. Accordingly one must help them as would Christ, Whom one really helps in helping them. . . . Yet let the sick also remember that one helps them for God's sake, and therefore let them not distress the nursing brothers with excessive demands. Also one must patiently bear with them, in this way one gains greater merit. Let it also be the chief care of the abbot that they shall not be neglected at any single point.' By the year 742 a Church Council is found requiring that 'all monks and nuns must organize and run their monasteries or hospitals according to the Rule of St. Benedict, and they shall themselves live according to this rule'.

The model for a group of hospital buildings is prescribed and the procedures to be followed are set out. In the building plans for any monastery provision was to be made for an *infirmarium*. This was, of course, primarily for the monks who became ill, but in the larger monasteries there was also a separate building eventually called 'the hospital' into which sick pilgrims and the seriously ill from the neighbourhood could be received. There was also in most cases what might be called an outpatients' room for pilgrims and the sick of the local community, together with a separate hospice for travellers. Each monastery had its herb garden where medicinal plants such as cumin, fennel, mint, rosemary, rue and sage were grown for their therapeutic properties, as well as for culinary use. Charlemagne is reported to have kept his own herb garden. One was attached to all, or most, of the important religious communities in Central Europe, such as those at Bobbio (Pavia), St. Rupert (Salzburg), St. Kilian (Würzburg) and Reichenau (Lake Constance).

In Britain a number of such infirmaries, hospices, elementary 'hospitals' and herb gardens were established, for example at St. Columba's, Iona (563) and St. Cuthbert's, Lindisfarne (635). Missionaries from Britain to the Continent also founded cloister schools, hospices, and hospitals, notably Boniface at Fulda, and Alcuin and Fulbert at Tours.

One of the best known hospitals in Europe was established by Bishop Masona in 580 at Merida in Spain. It was described as a 'large hospital'. From it came several case reports which show signs of progress in medical knowledge, including an account of certain surgical procedures which are unexpected at these early dates. Similar hospitals were founded in each of the succeeding centuries, and among those for which most information is available are St. John the Almsgiver at Ephesus (founded about 610), the Hôtel Dieu at Paris (where a start seems to have been made by the Bishop of Paris in 651, though the first full historical record is dated 829), Montpellier (738), St. Albans (794), St. Maria della Scale, Siena (898), St. Conrad's, Constance (968) and St. Bernard's Hospice in the Swiss Alps (962).

PERIOD 3: THE MEDIEVAL HOSPITALS (1000-1500)

On coming to the Middle Ages — especially in the 12th century — we find that the number of hospitals greatly increased. In cities with large Christian populations there were moves to provide on a bigger scale both hospices for travellers and hospitals for the sick. In some countries the number of these new foundations is quite surprising.

The new institutions were of two kinds. The first were basically an expansion of the services already provided in earlier centuries by the monastic infirmaries. When an increasing number of the monks 'professed' medicine and began to extend their attentions to the local population and to the travellers in the hospices, there was a considerable increase in the need for more hospital accommodation and a growth in the number of wards required to receive the seriously ill from around the monastery. Secondly, in cathedral cities and large towns there were moves to provide more public hospitals which would increasingly have the financial support of the city fathers. In these there was a new trend towards the appointment of *lay* physicians, especially after the Church placed a ban on monks practising outside of the monasteries, because it was considered to be interfering with the true nature of their spiritual calling. Beginning in a few prosperous centres, this movement grew until eventually few major cities or towns were without something of the kind.

Separate from both these types of institution were the many isolation hospitals for leprosy patients, for this was the period of the greatest incidence of this disease in Western Europe. At that time they were known as 'lazar houses', from the old French 'lazar' meaning 'leper' (derived from the name of Lazarus). From the findings of a French study for the period of the Hundred Years War, F. H. Garrison states that in England and Scotland there were more than 220 such 'lazar houses' and that there were '2,000 in France alone'! Most of the earliest pioneering activity in the founding of the lazar houses had come from the Church. It was not until the 13th and 14th centuries that the municipal authorities were clearly involved to any extent in the initiation and support of such institutions. When in the 14th and 15th centuries the incidence of leprosy became greatly reduced and had virtually ceased, some of these lazar houses were transferred to municipal and other authorities for other uses.

As already described (p. 11) the first monastic hospitals were modelled on the earliest foundation of the Benedictine Order at Monte Cassino. In Britain examples are to be found in the chief cathedral cities, such as the infirmary at St. Albans which was already active by A.D. 794. This was followed in 1118 by St. John's Hospital, Canterbury. Other later examples are the Holy Cross Hospital, Winchester, founded in 1132; St. Bartholomew's Hospital, London, in 1137; St. Thomas's Hospital, London, in 1215; and St. Mary's Spital, London, in 1179. The latter in 1247 became the hospital of St. Mary of Bethlem or 'Bedlam', and, in view of its subsequent history in psychiatry, it is interesting that it accepted mental cases from the beginning. There were many comparable new foundations on the Continent of Europe; one to achieve fame in the history of medical education was the Hospital of the Holy Ghost, built at Montpellier in 1145. It was to become an influential teaching centre.

However, the main period of Christian hospital building in the Middle Ages came in the 12th century. It was started and encouraged by Pope Innocent III, who in 1198 built the Santo Spirito Hospital in Rome. It led to a great wave of similar building. A monastic Order was specially founded with this aim and a Hospital of the Holy Ghost became established in virtually every major city. In most of the countries served by these hospitals the secular authorities were challenged and stimulated by the Church's example.

The first steps in providing for public health were undertaken, however, by some of the more enlightened city councils. For example, the appointment of a city physician for Bologna is recorded in the year 1214. He might be considered the prototype of the Medical Officers of Health of the 19th and 20th centuries and of the community physicians of today.

Making their influence felt in a number of ways were other new religious Orders. Several came into being at the time of the Crusades, for example the Order of St. John of Jerusalem (1099) and the (German) Order of St. Mary of the Teutonic Knights of Jerusalem (1198). The former were responsible for starting three efficient hospitals, the first in Jerusalem, the second on the island of Rhodes and the third in Malta. To this day the St. John's Hospital of the Knights in Malta is believed to possess the largest hospital ward in the world. It is said that it could comfortably take up to 150 patients at one time. Included in the vow taken by the Teutonic Knights was an undertaking to care for the sick and to build a hospital in whatever place they settled. It is, however, necessary to add here that the deterioration of the original motives of the Crusades and later developments in these military Orders took them far from the letter and spirit of the founders.

Supplementing the work of such men's Orders, and sometimes exceeding them in spiritual zeal, were comparable women's communities, for example the Sisters of St. Catherine of Siena, who introduced the beginnings of a regular nursing unit. The devoted women followers of St. Elizabeth of Hungary were similarly active. They were responsible for the building of two impressive hospitals at Eisenach.

THE LARGE NUMBER OF MEDIEVAL HOSPITALS

Throughout the three centuries, from the 13th into the 15th century, the founding of hospitals continued in Europe. In two carefully researched articles R. Virchow showed that in the 14th century the number of hospitals of the Holy Ghost rose impressively to 155 in the German cities. He also demonstrated that these were supplemented by a large number of lazar houses for leprosy victims. The process of hospital construction rose to its full height in the 15th century when there were many hospital buildings, such as those called Hôtel Dieu (God's Hospitality) or of the Santo Spirito type, in the majority of important European cities.

How many there were in England is not easy to assess because of the use of the word 'hospital' for institutions which aimed to meet other needs than those of the medical care of patients who were seriously ill. The term 'hospital' included institutions which were really 'hospices' for orphans, the destitute, the aged and poor elderly clergy. R. M. Clay in her *The Mediaeval Hospitals of England* has researched into the available charters and trust deeds of the medieval buildings called 'hospitals' in order to reveal the initial purpose of each of these foundations and their subsequent uses. She claims that in England alone there were nearly 800 institutions which used the name 'hospital'. Although the aims of a considerable number of these were wider, a good proportion were concerned with the needs of the sick.

During this period on the Continent there was a considerable growth of monastic type hospitals as a result of the activities of the Benedictines. At the time of the death of St. Benedict of Nursia in the sixth century there were 14 monasteries which were following his rule requiring special attention to and provision for the sick. Estimates for the number of Benedictine monastery hospitals which were active towards the end of the Middle Ages have been given in thousands. The number was certainly very large. Unlike their counterparts in England, their services in most countries of Europe were not immediately curtailed by the Reformation. There was a more gradual transfer of responsibility to public administration by the municipal authorities.

Though the advances in medical treatment during the Middle Ages seem to us so slow and meagre it is very clear that the various hospices and hospitals met a great social need. A measure of relief and mitigation of their suffering was brought to thousands of sick persons. It can be seen that to the limits of its knowledge, economic resources and practical possibilities the Christian Church had made an immense contribution to the medical needs of the communities it sought to serve.

PERIOD 4: HOSPITALS FROM 1500-1800

THE NEGATIVE EFFECTS OF THE REFORMATION

The suppression by royal authority of the monastic hospitals in England at first brought confusion and seeming disaster to many of the communities. For while it was responsible for bringing much spiritual good, some of the initial medical effects of the Reformation were less happy. In those countries where the monasteries were immediately suppressed, and the nursing sisterhoods curtailed in their work, there were two immediate effects. First, the loss of many of the monastery hospitals removed from many suffering and handicapped persons the only support they had. Then the disbanding of the brotherhoods and sisterhoods which had staffed the hospitals removed the local medical and nursing care from both the institutions and surrounding communities.

When in 1536-39 Henry VIII moved to take over the monasteries, his orders were carried through with considerable vigour and thoroughness. All the monastic properties and endowments passed to the Crown at first. The immediate effects were catastrophic, as for example, in the case of hospitals such as St. Bartholomew's and St. Thomas's in London. They were closed and their inmates virtually thrown on the streets. This lamentable situation lasted for some time until the City Fathers woke up to what they could do and Parliament was compelled to pass Acts for 'Poor Relief'.

The most favourable outcome of the situation was that it forced the civic authorities to pay increasing attention to the health problems of the community. In London those responsible for St. Bartholomew's Hospital approached the City Corporation, and the Lord Mayor eventually submitted a petition to Henry VIII for the refund to the hospital of its share of the monastic endowments, and for the transfer to the Corporation of the hospital's administration. After six years' delay Henry replied granting the main requests and refounding the hospital with the official title — 'The House of the Poor in West Smithfield of the Foundation of King Henry VIII'! He endowed it with the sum of 500 marks annually and required the City of London to match this by 500 marks annually and to maintain the buildings. The King also returned its endowments to St. Thomas's, which the City had bought, and changed the dedication to St. Thomas the Apostle instead of St. Thomas of Canterbury. The city had also bought the St. Mary of Bethlem Hospital, which continued to care for psychiatric patients.

These proved to be the only hospitals of importance to be refounded in England before the next hospital-building movement in the 18th century. There were, however, signs of an increase in the lay interest in medicine and hospital institutions which was later to bear fruit.

THE 18TH CENTURY REVIVAL OF HOSPITAL BUILDING

The 18th century brought to the British Isles great changes in the national outlook. In addition to the beginnings of social changes caused by the drift of the population from the country to the great industrial cities, there came the impact of new philosophic, scientific, and educational thought known in European history as 'the Enlightenment'. During the same period a widespread revival of religion took place as a result of the preaching of the evangelists John Wesley, George Whitefield and others, while the world of medicine benefited from the growth of a new philanthropic movement which powerfully aided those who were planning new ventures and helped to raise capital for their new hospital buildings and income for their maintenance.

So greatly did the number of hospitals increase at this time that it has been called the 'age of hospitals'. The majority of the new institutions were primarily for the 'sick poor' and were mainly supported by voluntary contributions. Historians agree that 'hospitals in the modern sense were certainly one of the effects of the Christian revolution . . . (which) introduced a new attitude to the sick, an attitude of pity and a desire to help which was quite new in that it extended to strangers and, still more remarkable, to the poor'. No technical advance in Medicine accounts for this expansion. Increase in population and the population shifts associated with urbanization could account for only a small part of it. It was the impact of the Gospel of Christ which affected the nation, both through lives dedicated to his service, and by their creating a movement of thought and behaviour in which deeds of mercy came naturally to Christian and non-Christian alike. More often than not it was deeply devout Christians who were the leading figures in the voluntary hospital movement. Anglicans, Nonconformists and Quakers alike were all involved.

PIONEER VOLUNTARY HOSPITALS IN ENGLAND

When Louis XIV revoked the Edict of Nantes in 1685, many French Protestants fled to England to escape persecution. In 1708 they founded a hospital in London for the poorer members of their community. Later this hospital ran short of funds and appeals for contributions were made so that it became in effect in the modern sense — the first 'voluntary' hospital in London. It limited its admissions to French Protestants (Huguenots), but nevertheless provided a pattern for the subsequent foundations in what soon became a widespread network of voluntary hospitals. Some of the earliest of these may be taken as examples of what was to be repeated constantly in London and other cities.

Westminster Hospital. In the early 18th century the only form of transport in London was by horse or horsedrawn vehicle along poorly made roads. London Bridge was the only bridge over the river. St. Thomas's Hospital was situated to the south of the river, roughly where London Bridge station now stands, while St. Bartholomew's Hospital lay to the north, near Smithfield. At this time the town of Westminster was increasing in population, but around it lay much low-lying marshland which was also liable to flooding. There were a number of other factors also which underlined the need for a local hospital at Westminster.

It was with such a background that a group of men met at St. Dunstan's coffee house on January 14, 1716 and produced 'a charitable proposal for relieving the sick and poor and other distressed persons', basing their project on the teaching of the parable of the Good Samaritan. Further discussions resulted in the opening of the Westminster Hospital in 1720 from which, later in the century, St. George's Hospital became an off-shoot. Among that group of men were Henry Hoare, 'a devout churchman'; William Wogan, 'a man of distinguished piety', who was the writer of many religious works and was on terms of friendship with Whitefield and Wesley; Robert Witham, biblical scholar and brother of Bishop George Witham; and Patrick Cockburn, a Scottish divine and writer of treatises on various aspects of the Christian faith.

The founder of *Guy's Hospital,* Thomas Guy, was a Baptist publisher who had succeeded financially. But, notwithstanding his wealth, he lived a spartan life. He is described as being 'truly charitable and did not wait until he was old and wealthy to give freely of what he had earned and saved'. In 1704 he became a governor of St. Thomas's Hospital, and became greatly concerned for the many patients who from time to time were discharged too weak and ill to earn a living. He therefore made provision in his will for the foundation of a hospital that was to bear his name and which would meet the needs of long-stay patients. His compassionate outlook is further illustrated by the fact that he sought also to make arrangements for the care of the chronically insane. When the new hospital was opened in 1726 it included a separate 'lunatic house' for 20 patients. This psychiatric department (in more modern forms) has continued into the present as a unit of Guy's Hospital.

The London Hospital was founded in 1740 by a surgeon, John Harrison. That he was prompted by Christian philanthropic motives is clear from the records and from his warm friendship with the Rev. Matthew Audley, who became chaplain of the hospital. The original constitution of the 'London' reads very much like that of an overseas mission hospital.

Prayers were to be read in the wards and patients on discharge were expected to go to thank Almighty God in their parish churches.

Highly significant in the progress of the voluntary hospital movement was the founding some years later of a medical school at the London Hospital by one of the surgeons there named William Blizzard. Surgeons had always tended to bring their apprentices into the wards of the hospital, but the establishment of a full medical school in London at that time was unique. It is clear that Blizzard's professional ability was remarkable. Appointed surgeon to the 'London' in 1780 he 'ranked with the giants' as an operator, and as a teacher he was quite outstanding. He performed his last operation — an above-knee amputation — when he was 84 years old, and even then 'his hand was as steady as at any period of his life'.

His Christian faith governed all that he did. One of the patients in his wards, who could read clearly, would be asked to read aloud a portion of Scripture at a convenient time each evening. In his concern for the under-privileged he founded a Samaritan Society which aimed to relieve the difficulties and distress of patients after they had left hospital.

In view of the fact that some religious people have not always adopted a sympathetic attitude to sexual problems, it is of interest to recall that the *London Lock Hospital* for the treatment of venereal diseases was founded in 1747 by a convert to Methodism.

THE PROVINCIAL CITIES

The 18th century hospital building period was by no means confined to London. Between the years 1736 and 1787 hospitals, mostly at this time called 'Infirmaries' were opened in 18 important cities. One of the earliest initiatives was taken in Cambridge by John Addenbrooke, a physician, who in 1719 left his large estate to provide a hospital for this university city. But Addenbrooke's Hospital did not open until 1766, just four years before the Radcliffe Infirmary in Oxford. Meanwhile, on October 28, 1736 the first patient had been admitted to the developing County Hospital at Winchester, which thus became the first of the provincial voluntary hospitals. The Rev. Alured Clark, prebendary of Winchester Cathedral, was a prime mover in this venture, having sought advice from the governors of Guy's and St. Thomas's Hospitals in London. The aim of the Winchester Hospital was 'to instruct the ignorant and reclaim the bad, while treatment of the physical disability was going on'. In 1741 Clark was transferred to Exeter where he became a co-founder of the Exeter Hospital (1743).

The beginning of the Royal Infirmary of Bristol followed hard on that of Winchester. The effective meeting of the Bristol planning committee took place in December 1736 and the building was opened to receive the first patient by the following December 1737. Northampton followed in 1743, Gloucester, Liverpool and Shrewsbury in 1745, Worcester in 1746 and Manchester in 1752, with others coming in gradually to cover the country.

In the majority of these cities the Church congregations and active Christians were well represented on the planning committees and were among the most energetic members of the Councils. For example, in Northampton, those mainly concerned were Philip Doddridge and Dr. (later Sir) James Stonehouse. Doddridge was the well-known Nonconformist divine, principal of a Nonconformist academy, and hymn writer, whose hymns are still sung today. Stonehouse had in early life been something of a cynic and had written an anti-Christian pamphlet. On coming to Northampton, however, he was converted through the influence of Doddridge and they worked actively together in the interests of the hospital project.

SCOTLAND

There had been a number of early initiatives in Scotland's medical history. For example, in 1494 a 'Mediciner' was added to the staff of St. Mary's College (University) of Aberdeen. This was probably the first appointment of an academic teacher of Medicine to a university in the British Isles. So again, in the 18th century, Scotland anticipated by a few years the hospital foundings in the South. An anonymous tract had circulated from the year 1721, which advocated the start of a hospital in Edinburgh for the due practice of Medicine and the task of restoring, where possible, incapacitated workers to their trades. In 1725 the Council of the Royal College of Physicians of Edinburgh agreed to support an appeal for funds to build an Infirmary. Christian philanthropy rose to the occasion and the first 18th century hospital in Scotland was opened in 1729, to become known as 'the Little Hospital in Robertson's Close'. The College of Physicians appointed two fellows 'to attend to the needs of the poor', presumably on an honorary basis. Glasgow followed with its

Town Hospital in 1733 and Aberdeen with the Infirmary in 1742. In view of Aberdeen University's original appointment of a 'Mediciner', it is interesting that from the first the Professor of Medicine there was permitted to bring his students on clinical visits to the Infirmary.

NORTH AMERICA

The first hospital in the United States was founded in Philadelphia by a Quaker, Thomas Bond. He had studied medicine in England, where he had become friendly with John Fothergill, also a Quaker (see p. 79). On returning to America, and seeing the prevalent illnesses for which there was little or no provision, Bond decided to establish a hospital for the reception and 'cure of poor sick persons'. His plan received the support of Benjamin Franklin and the hospital opened in 1751 with a Quaker widow as its first matron.

The Pennsylvania Hospital, Philadelphia, was founded on the same principles as its British voluntary hospital counterparts, especially those of St. George's and Winchester; but it differed from them in that it also provided private beds which were an attraction to the middle classes and brought some of its income. It also supplied the hospital facilities for the first American medical school. John Morgan, the first specialized physician, was behind this development and he became its first Professor of Physic. Bond's friend John Fothergill sent the new medical school a set of 'pretty accurate anatomical drawings, about half as big as the life', and these must have been valuable when subjects for dissection were hard to come by.

THE EUROPEAN CONTINENT

Limits of space prevent extensive reference to similar projects on the Continent, except for a mention of several social movements in the Churches of the 18th century. At the close of the Thirty Years War all public institutions in Central and Western Europe were at a low ebb. When recovery came the Churches in some countries, for example Switzerland, transferred their responsibility for medical and social welfare to the civic authorities. In other countries, such as the Netherlands and France, the Reformed Churches — having restored the order of deacons — gave them the responsibility to work for the sick, orphaned children and the alleviation of other social evils. The Reformed Churches of the Netherlands were especially admired for the efficient management of their orphanages.

Similarly in Germany the Pietists in the Lutheran Churches brought an infectious inspiration to the task and set an impressive example with their specialized institutions covering a variety of needs. Outstanding among them was the work of August Hermann Francke, a Lutheran parish minister and Professor of Greek in the University of Halle. A series of philanthropic institutions — including a successful pharmacy — grew up attached to his Church. At the time of his death there were 2200 children under his care and his staff included 175 teachers. At the same time he was giving free board to some 250 impecunious students of the University of Halle. Francke's example provided models for his 19th century successors in these forms of philanthropy, who included Theodore Fliedner of Kaiserswerth and George Müller of Bristol.

THE DISPENSARY MOVEMENT

Most hospitals of those days did not run an out-patient department (the Pennsylvania Hospital in the U.S.A. was an exception). To meet the widespread calls from the congested central areas of the large cities dispensaries were set up where physicians and poor patients could be brought into contact and from these buildings could visit the homes of the poor who were sick. Apart from such specialist advice, the patient depended on the local apothecary or 'chemist', who (in those days) was the prototype of the general practitioner. Such a dispensary had been opened in London by the Royal College of Physicians in the 17th century and more were set up in the 18th. By the 19th century, however, the emergence of hospital out-patients' departments rendered them mostly obsolete, except for the (Christian) Medical Missions in the underdoctored areas of some of the largest cities (p. 146).

The first dispensary specifically for small children was founded by George Armstrong, the son of a clergyman, in Red Lion Square, London. He later wrote a book on the diseases 'most incident to children'. A Quaker physician, John Coakley Lettsom, was the moving spirit behind the general dispensary which opened in 1770 in Aldersgate, London, with Dr. Nathaniel Hulme as its first physician. The latter was also the first librarian to the Medical Society of London and, in 1772, physician to the City of London Lying-In Hospital. Hulme was 'an amiable honourable

man of learning and scientific taste'. That he was an active Christian is
assumed from the publication in the *Gentleman's Magazine* of the full text
of his last prayer. John Wesley, the evangelist, who was constantly
concerned for the total welfare of those for whom he felt responsible,
opened a similar dispensary for the sick poor in 1746 in the City of London
near Wesley's Chapel. By 1800 there were in all some 14 dispensaries in
London.

These dispensaries were used not only for treatment, but also for the
teaching of medical students. When Robert Willan, the Yorkshire
Quaker and founding father of British dermatology, could not get a
hospital post because of his Nonconformist beliefs, he, together with his
assistant Thomas Bateman, worked and taught at the dispensary in Carey
Street.

PERIOD 5: THE 19TH AND 20TH CENTURIES

New voluntary hospitals were still being opened throughout the country
in the 19th and first part of the 20th centuries. Few cities and towns were
eventually left without one, and many small towns and large villages
came to possess their 'cottage hospitals'. But now there was a new development in the nature of some of these foundations. In step with the
increasing specialization among physicians and surgeons, some of the
new hospitals were planned to confine their attention to a particular
group of diseases. The process had begun in the middle of the 18th
century with the 'lying-in hospitals' which served the needs of the more
difficult maternity cases. A number of early steps were also taken to help
sick deserted and destitute children.

In 1725 John Maubray called attention to the services to mothers provided by the Hôtel Dieu of Paris, with its beginnings of a maternity
department and a school for midwives. He appealed for 'Christian
charity' to make similar arrangements in England. The first practical step,
however, was taken by a surgeon in Dublin, Bartholomew Mosse, who
established in 1745 the 'Dublin Lying-In Hospital' (subsequently in 1767
called the 'Rotunda', from the shape of part of the new buildings). While
'Christian charity' no doubt had to be relied on for this occasion — as
many of the pioneers increasingly had to do — Mosse resorted to new
channels to obtain support from the wealthier citizens. With the increase
in numbers of new hospitals, raising money for the voluntary system
became something of a professional activity!

The first hospital provision in London for maternity care was the result of the initiative of Richard Manningham, son of the Bishop of Chichester. He leased the house next to his own in Jermyn Street and in 1739 opened a small nursing home of 25 beds for obstetrics. The first of the London general hospitals to allocate a ward to such cases was the Middlesex Hospital. But there was some reluctance among the Governors to continue this course because of costs. In 1749 some of the Middlesex Hospital gynaecologists, with others, opened a small lying-in hospital of 20 beds, which developed later into the well-known Queen Charlotte's Hospital. These beginnings gave birth to a series of similar projects and between 1745 and 1913 (when the Mothers' Hospital was opened at Clapton by the Salvation Army) twenty-six major maternity hospitals were opened in the British Isles, besides many more small local ones serving limited areas.

All too belatedly steps were also taken in the interests of suffering children. In 1741 a retired seafarer, Thomas Coram, after vigorous appeals for funds (assisted by Hogarth the painter), opened the Foundlings Hospital — for orphaned and destitute children — on an ideal site north of Bloomsbury in London. A second major step in London was taken by a physician, John Bunnell Davis, who appealed for 'the support of Christian charity' in his efforts to establish a 'Universal Dispensary for Sick and Indigent Children'. It was started in 1816 and for over 50 years treated a large number of children. By this date a number of such children's hospitals had already come into being in some of the cities of the Continent. One had also been established in Manchester.

Because of the increasing number of difficult domicilary visits, it was not long before the staff of Davis' Children's Dispensary became convinced of the need for in-patient care. A few hesitant and amateurish steps were taken by the Committee to attach a ward to the Dispensary so that a small 'Infirmary' took shape. In 1839 a young physician, Charles West, was introduced to it. He had trained at St. Bartholomew's Hospital, London and the Rotunda in Dublin. He was specially interested both in midwifery and child health. Son of a Baptist minister he entered on this project with zeal. In 1842 he was appointed physician to the Children's Dispensary and by 1846 was agitating for the Infirmary to be considerably enlarged on its Waterloo Road site. The Committee, however, proved too lukewarm, or inept, in the task of raising sufficient new financial help to alter the position and Charles West resigned. He became lecturer in Medicine at the Middlesex Hospital, where he produced his *Lectures on Diseases of Infancy and Childhood* (in the third 1854 edition of which is a new chapter devoted to the disorders of the mind in childhood, one of the first of its kind).

In spite of his resignation from the Dispensary and its Infirmary, West was still very much concerned with the practical needs of children. One evening in June 1849 he took a walk northwards through Lincoln's Inn Fields and passed the former residence of the well known 17th century physician Dr. Phillip Mead. An inspiration suddenly came to him to found a children's hospital on that site. He succeeded in interesting other physicians and new supporters, and eventually 49 Great Ormond Street was leased for twenty-one years as the site for a children's hospital. To gain ideas and experience West soon began to take further steps in the interests of his child patients and was responsible for opening children's convalescent homes in the rural districts of Highgate and Mitcham. In 1865 he also pioneered a home and school for delicate and asthmatic boys on the coast at Bournemouth.

THE BACKGROUND

The Christian inspiration which was responsible for the origin of many of the hospitals is well illustrated by the beginnings of the Fever Hospital, King's College Hospital, the Royal Free Hospital and the Royal Marsden Hospital.

By 1800 there were already fever hospitals in Chester, Dublin, Liverpool and Manchester. London had none. Due to the overcrowded tenements and lack of sanitation such a provision was necessary, for the infectious cases could not gain admission to the general hospitals. At this time that remarkable philanthropic group of evangelical Anglicans, the Clapham Sect, with their base at Clapham Common, were already entering the field at various points, for example, with their Society for the Betterment of Conditions of the Poor. Among them were such reformers as William Wilberforce and Shute Barrington, Bishop of Durham. When the need for isolation became clear they promptly formed a Committee — in which Wilberforce and Barrington were included — and in 1802 opened the London Fever Hospital. The medical side was represented by the active Quaker philanthropist and physician John Coakley Lettsom (p. 80).

The Hospital continued in operation until the advent of the National Health Service when it was merged with the Royal Free Hospital group.

King's College Hospital was founded in 1840. The College in the Strand had been established in 1828 and the medical faculty was added to it in 1831. The project for the college came from the Rev. George D'Oyly, chaplain to the Archbishop of Canterbury, through whom the patronage of King George IV was obtained. The University of London, as University College, had in 1826 been founded on a secular basis. The basic principle for King's College was that 'every system of general education for the youth of a Christian community ought to comprise instruction in the Christian religion as an indispensable part'. Similar ideals lay behind the new medical school. 'In establishing a school of Medicine and Surgery in King's College, the Council has been influenced by the belief that many individuals who intend their sons for the Medical Profession will gladly embrace an opportunity of placing them in connexion with an institution which has for its principal object to educate the rising generation in the doctrines of Christianity, as taught by the Established Church, and to fix in their minds the true principles of morality.' The new medical school took over St. Clement Danes Workhouse and opened it as a fifty-bedded hospital for the relief of the sick poor. It was to be supported by voluntary contributions, and clinical medical students from King's College were to have access to its beds. Within three months the number of beds was increased to 120.

The Royal Free and Marsden Hospitals. In early years the administration of most of the new hospitals was in the hands of boards of governors, whose members were appointed because they had agreed to give a certain minimum annual contribution. This gave them the right to provide letters of introduction to patients who wished to present themselves to the hospital for treatment either as in-patients or out-patients. Dr. William Marsden, who had been a pupil of Abernethy, was returning to his home one evening in 1827 when he found a girl lying desperately ill on the steps of a church. He found that she had been refused admission to St. Bartholomew's Hospital because she had neither a letter from a governor nor any money. Marsden — a sincere Christian man — was much moved by the girl's plight. He befriended her and subsequently founded a dispensary to treat the poor where such formalities were not required. During the London cholera epidemic this dispensary dealt with many victims at a time when the general London hospitals were refusing to admit any cases for fear of infection. In 1843 he moved the dispensary to a site in Grays Inn Road and built a hospital in association with it. This developed into the Royal Free Hospital, 'free' because it admitted patients without letters of introduction or deposits of money. In 1851 William Marsden also took over a small house in Cannon Row, West-

minster, for the reception of patients suffering from cancer. The home
was later moved to Brompton where it became the Royal Cancer
Hospital, and was subsequently renamed the Royal Marsden Hospital.

THE FIFTH AND FINAL PHASE

The building of large numbers of various types of voluntary hospitals,
which had dominated the 18th and 19th centuries, came to its climax in
the early years of the 20th century. Thereafter, while a few large general
hospitals were established, the majority of new foundations were of a
more specialized kind. It is broadly true to claim that up to 1948, when
under the National Health Service Act most of the voluntary hospitals
were taken over by the State, a high proportion of their financial support
had come from the Churches and individual Christian philanthropists. It
was not just a matter of holding regular 'Hospital Sundays' in the
churches, sermons in aid of the hospitals and collections at church
services. Nor was it simply the task of recruiting from churches and
Christian organizations the personnel to carry out 'flag day' collections
and other special fund-raising measures, such as Alexandra's Rose Day
for the Children's Hospitals. For when Appeals Secretaries of the
hospitals masterminded on a grand scale approaches to the wealthy and
successful businessmen, their lists tended to concentrate on those most
suspected of being Christian philanthropists!

It is true that the large sums eventually obtained were a tribute to the
generosity of the total general public and new support from many other
quarters, but it seems certain that the voluntary system could not have
lasted as long as it did without the general Christian support it received.

There were several other ways in which the hospitals were indebted to
the churches. As will be illustrated in the story of the nursing profession
in Chapter 10, the difficult task of finding the thousands of nurses,
therapists and members of other ancillary services, which were required
to staff the large institutions growing up across the country, once again
tested Christian resources. The centuries old tradition of the women's
nursing orders in the Middle Ages was succeeded by the new armies of
trained nurses and other workers of the 20th century's health services.
Prominent Christian leaders have assisted from time to time in their
recruitment by making clear to their congregations that they regarded the
medical profession, the nursing profession, and medical missions as
appropriate channels into which their Christian ideals might be

channelled.   The debt owed by the voluntary hospitals to Christian support over the centuries is beyond computation.

CHAPTER 3

PRESERVING PAST GAINS AND PROGRESS

THROUGHOUT antiquity a practical difficulty confronting any school of thought was continuity and the preservation of its basic teachings. It was not only the human labour required regularly to copy the manuscripts but, in those unsettled and dangerous times, the preservation of important records from physical deterioration or destruction by invader or vandals. Until the invention of printing ensured adequate duplication of a new book, there was always the risk that the manuscripts — particularly of the works of less known authors — would be lost.

For Medicine this consideration was of increasing importance. Both in the Western and the Eastern parts of the Roman Empire the medical workers were still largely dependent upon treatises from the ancient Greek schools of medicine, represented either by the traditional school of Hippocrates from classical times or by the later school of Galen. At that period in history a number of factors combined to make the Christian communities, especially the monasteries with their libraries, the main custodians of much of the existing medical literature.

One particular feature in the organization of the Empire that simplified communications among the Christians was that the Greek language was still used over vast areas, notably in Asia Minor, the Near East and Egypt. Surprisingly, it remained also the dominant language in Southern Italy and was even used by a minority in Rome itself. This had the advantage that the Christian communities were in contact with Greek civilization, especially with the best of its legacy in Medicine, and Christian doctors, such as there were, tended to be well informed concerning the traditional Greek schools of thought. The Christian theological leaders were at first suspicious of Greek Medicine because of its pagan background and its use of incantations. There was later to be a practical compromise with this and several other traditions.

THE FALL OF ROME

The fall of the city of Rome marked the end of an era for the Western part of the Roman Empire. The Visigoths and other Teutonic peoples swept across the frontiers and began to consolidate their gains. By the time Theodoric the Great (455-526) became King of the Ostrogoths it was clear that they had come to stay. Much of great value in the literary and art treasures of Greece and Rome was lost during the ceaseless raids and wars. The newcomers — basically nomadic and pastoral peoples — set up a new style of empire which had little use for what remained of the classical heritage of the West. It was now the turn of the Eastern (Byzantine) part of the Roman Empire to preserve what it could of the earlier culture, and this to some extent it did until the eighth and ninth centuries when the Muslim Arabic-speaking armies pressed ever more heavily upon it. Eventually Egypt, North Africa and Spain were overrun in turn, and the spread of the Arab armies over the Pyrenees into France was not halted until the crucial battle near Tours in 732. The city of Byzantium itself held on, with some of its central territory intact, until the end of the Middle Ages.

However, with the rise of Charlemagne (742-814) at the head of the empire of the Franks in Central and Western Europe, some of the advantages of the earlier civilization were to be restored, a recovery in which the Christian Church was destined to play a worthy part. Even so, from the year 732 until well into the medieval period after 1100, Medicine at its best was mostly to be found among the Arabic-speaking doctors of the Near East, North Africa and Spain. Much later there was to be renewed progress in the West. Starting at Salerno (where there is evidence of a medical school as early as 856, and certainly from 946) the two traditions, Byzantine and Arabic, were eventually merged in the late 11th century to give rise to new developments during the later Middle Ages.

PRESERVING THE RECORDS

Shortly after the rise of the monastery founded in 529 by St. Benedict at Monte Cassino (see p. 11), its activities were turned into new channels by an industrious convert to Christianity, Aurelius Cassiodorus. He had served with distinction as Theodoric's chancellor and retired early in order to devote the rest of his life to good works — a service which he continued for some 25 years. In 540, on his own estate near Squillace he founded a new monastery to which he attached a hospital in accordance with the Benedictine rule. He also added a third institution, a medical school. He is known to have established other monasteries and hospitals along the trade routes and main places of pilgrimage. These hospitals frequently had elementary teaching units. It is from one such monastic medical school established by Cassiodorus at Benevente that our knowledge has been gleaned of the rules, the teaching curriculum and methods of the monastic communities which engaged in the service of the sick. Benevente was distinguished by a particular style of writing used in its manuscripts known as the 'beneventian script'.

A major part of the regular daily work of all these monasteries was the copying of medical and religious manuscripts. Where these were in Greek, as many were, they were frequently also translated into Latin. The extreme southern part of Italy was largely Greek-speaking, so that the monastic communities in that region were well equipped for this work and it was natural for them to endeavour to preserve the Greek *medical* manuscripts. The writings which the monastic schools were specially interested to preserve were those of Hippocrates, Soranus, Rufus of Ephesus, Aretaeus, Discorides and Galen. The Latin works which are mostly mentioned in any list are those of Celsus, Scribonus Largus, parts of Pliny the Elder and Caelius Aurelianus. This would be an average catalogue for the orthodox medical libraries of Italy of those times.

Copies of the Greek medical manuscripts, and/or their translations into Latin, seem to have found their way from such centres as Monte Cassino to the monasteries in other countries. F. H. Garrison comments that 'the *Encyclopaedia Physica* of the Abbot of Fulda, who was also Archbishop of Mainz (Hrabanus Maurus, Alcuin's favourite pupil and known as *primus praeceptor Germaniae,* 'the first teacher of the Germans') treats of medicine in the 6th, 7th and 18th books and gives a German-Latin glossary of anatomic terms'.

THE STANDARDS REACHED

Throughout this era medical teaching seems to have followed orthodox Greek Medicine with only marginal advances, except that some of the ablest practitioners took empirical steps forward in their practice of therapeutics. The general literature which has survived from the ancient libraries does not encourage the reader to expect much significant technical advance. For example, the knowledge of anatomy and physiology continued in a static 'orthodox' form, which was usually a Christian intepretation of the views of Galen. The manuscripts offering the Hippocratic and Galenic traditions continued to be accepted as valid in their details without much modification by clinical observation. Also, in the monastic hospitals much of the treatment was by spiritual procedures such as intercessory prayer, the laying on of hands and exorcism of evil spirits. One disadvantage of the passing of Medicine into the hands of the priest-physicians long continued to be felt. Procedures which could have favoured basic research, for example dissection of the human body or postmortem examinations, were for long ruled out by the ecclesiastical authorities on the ground that the body had been created in 'the image of God' and should not be violated. Except, however, for the Alexandrian school the same is true of both the pagans and the Arabic school. There are several other justifications for the complaint that in the Dark and Middle Ages the Christian influence on Medicine tended to delay scientific and medical advances.

It is all too easy, with the advantage of hindsight and the present state of our knowledge, to criticize failure to progress. It is now clear that the inherited traditions and their contemporary applications were often ineffectual and sometimes crude. The proffered remedy could be worse than the disease. There were good grounds, therefore, for Christian leaders to warn those who consulted non-Christian doctors about the dangers of therapeutic practices current at that time. For example, Pope Gregory complained: 'What can these doctors do with their instruments? It is more their concern to cause than to relieve pain. When they open the eye and cut into it with their sharp lancet, they make the patient suffer agonies in any case before they help him to see again. And as soon as some precautionary measures are not followed, it is generally a case of loss of their eyesight. Our dear Saviour on the other hand has only one instrument, His will, and only one salve, His healing power.' Today, cushioned by modern anaesthesia and increasing skills in surgery, a modern observer cannot make a truly realistic assessment of the position for both doctor and patient in the Dark Ages.

There were, however, two ways in which the priest-physicians gave welcome and often indispensable service, and also provided a salutary example in the treatment of the seriously ill. During the ancient pagan times even Hippocrates is said to have excused a physician who withdrew his services from a hopeless terminal case or from a seriously wounded enemy. The Christians, on the other hand, made it a point of honour to attempt to serve them, if possible to abolish pain, and to nurse them right to the end. Also, the priest-physicians, helped by residents from the religious communities, gave their services freely to the poor. Similarly, the Christian private practitioner (where he existed) was exhorted by the Church to be moderate and compassionate when charging fees.

PROGRESS THROUGH INDIVIDUALS

From this whole period, by the nature of the circumstances, only a few names of outstanding Christian practitioners have been preserved. One who clearly deserves further mention is Aurelius Cassiodorus. As has already been described, he led the members of Monte Cassino and his own monastic community at Squillace into new channels. He built what eventually became a large library, especially rich in manuscripts bearing upon the study of Science and Medicine. He was able to circulate many copies of the Greek writings (and their Latin translations) to other monasteries, and it was he who largely brought together the Greek, Latin and other traditions for the benefit of the later Middle Ages.

Another pioneer was Aëtius of Amida, a town in the Eastern Empire situated on the River Tigris. Aëtius was the royal physician to Justinian I, and from the way he writes, and the way in which Christian sacred names replaced the pagan ones in the charms which he uses, he appears to have been Christian at least in sympathy. He wrote a large book, the *Tetra Biblion,* in which he collected detailed records of the surgery, gynaecology and obstetrics of his day, together with accurate descriptions of epidemic diphtheria and other infectious diseases, as well as ear, nose and throat conditions. He also compiled what is believed to have been the first complete treatise on ophthalmology. His work also shows the beginning of independent clinical observations.

Another medical practitioner whose work has attracted the interest of historians is Alexander of Tralles. He was the brother of the Christian architect who rebuilt St. Sophia's Church in Constantinople and who, it is believed, first introduced to the world the construction of the dome. On several grounds Alexander himself is believed to have been a Christian, practising in the city of Rome where his professional opinion was respected and his treatment much sought after. He completed a 'system of medicine' in a series of 12 books. Although, like all writers of the time, he continues to show the usual deference to Galen, he does not follow him slavishly but expresses his own findings. Historians find clear evidence that much of his writing was based on observation and clinical experience. He wrote with care, paying tribute to Hippocrates and others when he had drawn upon their work, while expressing his own views where appropriate.

A further outstanding Byzantine writer was Paul of Aegina of the Alexandrian school of medicine. From a number of treatises which he is known to have written, only his seven volume work *On Medicine* survives.

It is the sixth of these volumes, *On Surgery,* which has aroused most interest. Its very accurate descriptions of surgical conditions and procedures enable historians to measure the extent of progress since Celsus. The *practical* skills of the surgeons had considerably advanced in spite of deficiencies in the contemporary knowledge of anatomy and physiology.

Besides evidences of originality in some of the individual writers, there are also signs of progress in medical training and the ways in which the best of the older traditions were being adapted. For example, Charlemagne sought to get the doctors of his day to merge the best from the classical Graeco-Roman tradition more fully with the Christian approaches of the monastic priest-physicians. With this in view he brought to Tours Peter of Pisa and his favourite scholar Alcuin of York and instructed them to revise the medical curriculum.

THE IMPROVEMENT OF ARABIC MEDICINE

At the beginning of the Middle Ages the services of Christians to Medicine were destined to have far-reaching and international effects in other directions. It is an interesting fact that it was largely through the Nestorian Christians (see p. 35) that the Arab world came to have accurate translations of the Greek and Byzantine medical books.

One of the ironies of history is that the conquerors of Egypt and North Africa soon came to regret their wanton destruction of the libraries of the West, especially that of the great library at Alexandria which was ruined by the Arab general Amrou in 638 when he sent many of the manuscripts to be used as fuel for the city's heating. They had special cause to deplore the loss of this library's scientific sections and paid heavily in an effort to recover copies of the lost treasures.

Early in the eighth century, Almansur, the Caliph of Baghdad, determined that the Arabic-speaking world should secure access to all the learning of the West, and in particular the best of the practical sciences, including Medicine. He therefore despatched emissaries with instructions to search for and acquire whatever Greek and Latin writings could be found. Where they were unable to buy copies of the works, copies were to be made and the translators handsomely paid to complete them. For over 100 years the cultural records of the West, especially the Greek writings, were in this way translated into Arabic. As a consequence Arab doctors were for 300 years at the growing points of study especially in Mathematics and Medicine.

In contrast with modern times, one feature of the administrations in the earliest Arabic Empires was their tolerance of racial, cultural and religious minorities and their openness to interchange. The result was that Christians and Jews were free to practise their religions and were employed by the Arab conquerors in the task of translation and the exchange of knowledge. These communities were particularly useful to them in these new quests because it gave them access to Greek and Roman thought. The Christians often had an accurate knowledge of Syriac, Arabic, Greek, Latin and sometimes Persian. Hence it was mainly the Christians and the Jews who were responsible for the great advances which took place in Arabic culture by the borrowing from the West. It accounts also for the prominent place which a number of both Christians and Jewish physicians came to occupy in the Arab world.

THE NESTORIAN CHRISTIANS

By far the greatest contribution to these tasks of translation was undertaken by the Nestorian Christians and by one of their families in particular. The founder of this Eastern sect, Nestorius, had to a large extent departed from orthodox Christianity and been deposed from the patriarchy of Constantinople. He sought to combine the teachings of the Christian faith as far as possible with those of Greek philosophy. The result was that, *culturally,* the Nestorians were among those best fitted to translate accurately and to ensure that details and nuances of Greek literature were conveyed in the Arabic. It also explains how a leading Caliph came to appoint a prominent Nestorian Christian, Ibn Mosawaih, to be the principal of his Baghdad school of scholars.

It was in such circumstances that the members of the Nestorian family of Bakhtichua (literally meaning 'servant of Jesus') were the chief Christian interpreters and translators for several generations and, also, gave a succession of court physicians to the Caliphs, continuing into the 11th century. In the first instance it was George (Jurjis) Bakhtichua, at that time medical director of the Nestorians' hospital and head of the medical faculty of the academy at Gondishapur, who was called to Baghdad by the Caliph. He was pressed to start translating the Greek medical writers and to plan the translation of all worthwhile medical authors whose works were still available. He had himself completed the translations of Hippocrates and Discorides before a serious illness overtook him. His son succeeded him in the task and also became a famous court physician, being in turn succeeded by members of his family as both translators and physicians.

Other Christians, such as John Masué the Elder, Serapion the Elder and Salmouih ben Bayan also took part in this important work of translation or became distinguished physicians in the Arabic Empire. The influence of the Nestorians extended to the adjoining lands of the Near East. They built several efficiently run hospitals in these countries, including a large and important one in the Khorassan province of Southwest Persia.

ARABIC MEDICINE

The scope of this study does not permit further reference to the 300 years of the rise and accomplishments of the Arabic School of Medicine, culminating in such names as Rhazes, Haly ben Abbas, Avicenna and Averroes. Nor is there room to pay due tribute to the part played by Jewish doctors in the Arabic renaissance, culminating in the work of physicians such as Maimonides. The fact that Rhazes, ben Abbas and Avicenna were Persians shows how open the Arabic world of that time was to receive help from outside.

The Arabic-Jewish-Christian era in Medicine was not, however, a time of blind acceptance of the Graeco-Roman, Jewish or Christian traditions. The Arabs themselves made significant additions to knowledge and students flocked to the great Arabic hospitals and to the medical teaching centres such as those at Baghdad, Damascus and Cordova. The Arabic medical schools also became rich in their library resources and each developed a flourishing herb garden. It is relevant to add that, at least in the period of their early development, the Arabic hospitals admitted patients without respect of religion, race or social rank.

THE RETURN OF MEDICINE TO THE WEST

During the next phase of medical development the West was to receive back from the Near East and North Africa its heritage in a new and enhanced form. The total gain from this return of medical knowledge from the East to the West was not just the reception of the old Greek Medicine in Saracen dress. The Arabic and Persian doctors had added a number of new substances, including chemicals, to the materia medica. The word 'drug' is of Arabic origin and the value of camphor, laudanum and senna were discovered by Arabic doctors. Also, it was in Baghdad that the division first became apparent between physicians, pharmaceutical botanists and apothecaries (called *Sandalani* in Arabic because they also bought and sold sandalwood). While surgery as a whole made little progress in the Arabic world, their ophthalmologists were at that time far ahead of those in the other countries.

From an academic point of view the return of the medical leadership to Western Europe came at a favourable time. For the Church was now actively promoting moves for the founding of a *studium generale* (university), and in most cases more than one in each country of the West. Soon after their opening the majority of the universities added a Faculty of Medicine. Indeed, several were themselves an extension of what, up till then, had been a successful medical school. As a result, this university movement eventually came to have a salutary influence on the future of Medicine.

One effect of the new university status on the practice and teaching of Medicine was that the Church's monastic hospital facilities were supplemented by the work of the university medical staffs and richer libraries. Eventually the process went far in gradually replacing the priest-physicians. Another effect was the beginning – or perhaps the hastening – of a trend towards the secularization of the medical profession. In several ways this had its good side in that the empirical approach and the beginnings of experimental science (as applied to Medicine) among the academic laymen led to advances in diagnosis and treatment. On the other hand, from the Church point of view, it posed a growing threat to the ecclesiastical discipline with which the daily practice of the profession had been guided and in future it would become orientated more towards lay organization and control. It heralded the beginning of a tension between Church, Science and Medicine in Europe which would in more modern times give some substance to the Jesuit dictum – 'Ubi tres medici, ibi duo athei' (where there are three doctors, two of them are atheists). At this time, however, the university medical faculties were mostly examples of further Christian initiatives and attempts to raise standards.

SALERNO

The prototype for the medieval university medical faculties emerged at Salerno in Southern Italy. A small medical school, attached to a monastic infirmary for pilgrims, had already existed there since the ninth century. It was not, however, until the middle of the 11th century that it came to have its greatest influence as a teaching centre. This crucial step came through the arrival in Salerno in 1065 of Constantine the African from North Africa. Constantine had been a merchant and during his travels had acquired an extensive knowledge of both Arabic and Classical Medicine. He was converted to Christianity and, later, in 1070 became a monk at the monastery of Monte Cassino. Here he devoted the remaining 17 years of his life to the collection and translation into Latin of works from both Greek Classical and Arabic Medicine.

The teachers at Salerno were among the first of the contemporary medical staffs of the West to benefit from the influences of Arabic Medicine. They set up a comprehensive curriculum based on the best to be found in the Greek and Arabic traditions. They probably also had other contacts with Arabic Medicine through some Jewish doctors who were working in their town.

While the medical school at Salerno was loosely under the influence of the Church authorities from Monte Cassino, it had an advantage over its rivals. Its growth is said to have come from a group of medical men themselves in pursuit of their professional interests in this health resort. Both its clientele and staff were cosmopolitan. Tradition has it that the pioneers of progress were four local practitioners of different races and religions — a Greek, a Roman, a Saracen and a Jew, each of whom is said to have taught the students in his own language. These 'doctors of Salerno' are believed to have formed themselves into a *collegium Hippocraticum* and to have gone on to develop a high standard of teaching which increasingly attracted students from other parts of Europe.

Bedside as well as theoretical instruction was given, and throughout the course there was regular basic teaching of anatomy. Some measure of scientific progress was achieved in most branches of Medicine, particularly high standards being reached in obstetrics and gynaecology. The latter department seems to have been taught and served by women doctors. Though several historians have taken the view that the names of women recorded refer to a superior type of midwife, the full evidence seems to leave little doubt that there were women doctors on the teaching staff and women medical students.

Several influential books came from this college. The best known was a very long Latin poem presenting a series of wise regulations and suggestions for dietary and personal hygiene — the *Regimen Sanitatis Salernitarum* (Rules of Health of the School of Salerno). It is said to have gone into 140 editions and to have been translated into many languages. It begins with a statement that it had been written for the 'King of the English', though it would appear that this mistakenly referred to Robert, Duke of Normandy (brother of William I), who had been wounded in the Crusades and recuperated at Salerno.

THE UNIVERSITY OF MONTPELLIER

A second important teaching centre developing during this period was the medical faculty of the University of Montpellier in Southern France. Indications of medical activity in this place are recorded as early as the year 738 when a clinic staffed by doctors of several races attracted a few students from other lands. Then four centuries later the Bishop of Mainz wrote of a series of instructive medical lectures which had been given at Montpellier in 1137. The chief account of professional instruction there, however, comes from details of a reorganization of the faculty by William IV in 1180-81. The aim was to end tension between Christian and Jewish physicians — the former followed the teaching of Salerno and the latter exclusively that of Arabic Medicine. A group of Jewish physicians had been active for some years in Montpellier, and rivalry with those of other outlooks had grown both in the local practices and on the teaching faculty. The eventual outcome of William IV's intervention, however, was that the curriculum of Salerno became recognized as that for 'a School of Medical Science': that is, it gave it university status.

On the faculty at Montpellier any qualified graduate in Medicine was permitted freely to lecture, whatever his views, religion and background. Montpellier University was not recognized by the Pope as a *studium generale* and so was not given full university status until 1289. Even then, however, when more directly under the authority of the Church, Montpellier continued to enjoy a certain degree of independence. In later years some of Europe's outstanding physicians were to receive their post-graduate education there.

OTHER NEW UNIVERSITIES

The great Christian movement for founding universities, which indirectly helped progress in Medicine, continued steadily over the next 300 years. During this period a succession of Popes recognized as a *studium generale* the teaching centres in some 47 cities of Western Europe, including those at Paris (1110), Bologna (1158), Oxford (1167), Cambridge (1209) and Padua (1222). In the majority of these universities medical faculties existed from the beginning or were soon established. This increase in the number of faculties undoubtedly raised the prestige of the medical graduates and teaching became more systematic. Examinations were introduced and had to be passed before a student could qualify and receive a licence to practise. There was greater unity and continuity in the handing on of the accepted body of teaching, while the university libraries preserved the writings of the masters of Medicine. The two university medical faculties which began to lead the way in the West were those of Paris and Bologna.

IMPROVED COMMUNICATIONS

In ways similar to the service performed by the Nestorian Christians in translating Greek and Byzantine medical writings into Arabic, and by Constantine the African and his followers at Monte Cassino (and Benevente) in bringing this heritage back to the West in an enhanced form, a general improvement in international communications was taking place. Gerard of Cremona translated into Latin some of the most important Arabic writings and was specially interested in the progress made by the Arabic 'eye doctors'. Roger of Palermo collected all that he could find of reliable work in surgery and in 1180 issued his *Post mundi fabricam* (the title taken from its opening words — 'After the Creation of the world'). It is believed to be the first textbook of surgery published in the Middle Ages. Subsequently under the title *Roger's Practice of Surgery* (as revised by one of his students, Rolando of Parma) it long remained in use as a major textbook.

However, the most original, practical and extensive of the textbooks of surgery (in five volumes) was that of William of Saliceto. It is a landmark in the history of surgery and introduces the beginnings of regional or surgical anatomy. William was an outstanding surgeon in 13th century Italy, and his genius spread into other fields as well. In 1275 he wrote another five-volume work which embraced all the important aspects of Medicine entitled *Summa Conservationis et Curationis* or *A Textbook of the Management and Cure of Sick Persons*. Holding the posts of Professor in the University of Bologna and, later, city medical officer of Verona, he worked incessantly to reconcile the two branches of the healing art — medicine and surgery — and to unite them in fruitful cooperation. He held advanced views on several surgical techniques, expressing doubt, for example, about the overfree use of the cautery (as practised by Arabic surgeons). He records his observations that wounds which had been treated with the cautery were more liable to suppuration than those treated with the knife. He taught that, ideally, wounds should heal by first intention and he himself used dressings of white of egg and rose water. He arrested haemorrhage by pressure and sutures. He was also ahead of his time in the diets he recommended, his regimen for personal hygiene and also his advocacy of isolation (and elementary forms of prophylaxis) for those suffering from infectious diseases.

Another surgeon who was in advance of his time was Theodore Borgognoni, a Dominican priest who became Bishop of Cerna. He was the son of Hugh of Lucca, who was one of the most skilled surgeons of those times. Borgognoni contended even more strongly than Saliceto that wounds should heal by first intention. The presence of 'laudable pus' was to be avoided; it was harmful and prevented the natural processes of healing. In a Lister-like manner he advocated the strictest cleanliness in all surgical techniques, including the thorough washing of the hands, and he discouraged the use of plasters and ointments. He himself washed a wound with wine before suturing the edges and dressed it with lint soaked in wine. In his book *Chirurgia* (not published until 1499) he confidently writes: 'It is not necessary, as Roger and Roland have written, as many other of their disciples declare and as all modern surgeons teach, that pus should be generated in a wound; no error can be greater than this. Such a process hinders nature, provokes the disease, and prevents the coagulation and consolidation of the wound.'

In all these respects he was followed by his distinguished pupil Henri de Mondeville who became court physician to Philip the Fair. Henri in his turn strenuously campaigned for the antiseptic (and a measure of aseptic) treatment of wounds, but he seems to have been the last in that century to do so. He taught the 'dry treatment' of wounds. He would wash the wound with wine and then put nothing on to it (such as the contemporary plasters and ointments), because he had observed that 'wounds dry much better before suppuration than after it'. In his treatise on surgery (*Cirurgia*), which he began to write in 1306, he offers much wise advice to surgeons which, had it been heeded and developed, would have led to valuable and timely progress. He became famous for such cutting remarks as 'many more surgeons know how to cause pus than to heal a wound' and 'God did not exhaust all His creative power in making a Galen'.

Another outstanding surgeon of the French school was Guy de Chauliac. After theological studies and ordination as a priest, he turned to the study of Medicine in Toulouse, Montpellier and Paris, and then followed a postgraduate course in anatomy in Bologna. He practised in the South of France and was physician to three popes during the 'captivity' at Avignon. From one point of view Chauliac put the clock back. He did not continue the 'dry treatment' of wounds or follow the first steps towards asepsis. On the other hand, he introduced beneficial reforms in the approach to operative surgery as a whole, especially for such common conditions as hernia and cataract. He believed in excision in cases of early cancer, but returned to the cautery for anthrax and advanced cancer. His advances in orthopaedics were considerable and he used sling bandages and weights for traction. His surgical textbook, *Inventorarium et Collectsorium* (1363) (later called *Chirurgia Magna,* or Textbook of Surgery) became the surgical *vade mecum* for many students and doctors in later generations. It is to Chauliac's lasting credit that, when most other doctors in his area fled in the plague years of 1348 and 1360, he stayed, sought to understand the infection and to devise some treatment for it.

THE CLOSE OF THE MIDDLE AGES

During the 13th, 14th and early 15th centuries, while there were a number of examples here and there of small advances by gifted individuals, the overall progress of Medicine was painfully slow. Small improvements were made in some surgical techniques and the more active of the physicians had minor successes. Arnold of Villanova, in his widely acclaimed pharmacopoeia, improved on a suggestion of Roger of Palermo. He found the value of burnt sponges and seaweed in the treatment of exophthalmic goitre, the first known therapeutic use of iodine. As a whole, however, the better days of medicine and surgery awaited the aftermath of the great intellectual and religious upheavals of the Renaissance and Reformation in which Christians of all viewpoints and professions were to be very much involved.

CHAPTER 4

EFFECTS OF THE NEW LEARNING

TOWARDS the late Middle Ages signs were not lacking of a radical change in the intellectual outlook and religion of the West. In all departments of life a new world order was struggling to be born. The process, however, was destined to be very slow, and it spread over more than a century. For the old order was deeply entrenched and neither the new learning, nor the new religion, were by any means welcomed by a reactionary medieval Church. Hence the influence of Christians became divided. As represented by the papal establishment it tended to delay or even obstruct some lines of advance. As represented by the new reformed Churches, however, it was in the vanguard of scientific progress. One important outcome was the liberation of Medicine from the monasteries and priest-physicians and the growth of an independent lay profession.

So far as the march of Medicine was concerned there were clearly both gains and losses. The Roman Church authorities, with their ban on the dissection of the human body, insistence on orthodox Medicine, and their suspicion of experiment, undoubtedly delayed the growth of the basic sciences as applied to Medicine. This was specially true of anatomy and physiology, which for long could not challenge the inaccuracies of the ancient authorities, whose knowledge was mainly based on dissection of animals. On the other hand, here and there gifted individual workers appeared, who all the time pressed forward with such light as they had. Some of these deserve appropriate mention.

THE DEVELOPMENT OF ANATOMY

Those concerned to build a more accurate knowledge of human anatomy and physiology had need of great courage and determination. For in those times to question Galen was to invite ridicule or opposition, and in the later years of the Middle Ages attracted the attention of the formidable Inquisition. It is therefore worthy of our respect that from the occasional dissection of a corpse (e.g. of an executed criminal, legally permitted to them, and of other cadavers dubiously acquired) some of the chief lecturers in anatomy were able to go as far as they did. Dissection of a human body and lecturing directly on anatomy seems first to have taken place in Bologna towards the beginning of the 13th century. By the time of William of Saliceto the surgeons showed an increased acquaintance with human anatomy and included aspects of surgical anatomy in their textbooks of surgery.

The first lecturing and writing in a full course of human anatomy is believed to have been by Henri de Mondeville in Montpellier, and more particularly as the course was developed by his colleague Mordino de Luzzi, usually known as Mundinus. De Mondeville had been a student at Bologna and brought with him to Montpellier the latest anatomical and surgical teaching, including the best from the Arabic tradition. His fellow member of staff, Mundinus, made a systematic study of the human body by careful dissection at the University of Montpellier. The latter's practical and complete textbook of anatomy, produced in 1316, is said to be the first volume of its kind in Europe. It includes not only anatomy but physiology, with a number of original practical observations. It also contains the beginnings of applied anatomy and applied physiology. Another important aspect of the work of Mundinus is that he did all the dissections himself and did not employ others in the menial tasks of the project. Also his work included the first major step towards the invaluable supplement of accurate illustration, which had to await the brighter days of Leonardo da Vinci and Vesalius for its completion.

THE 13TH CENTURY MINI-RENAISSANCE

In the general climate of opinion at this time four first class minds gave hope of better things. While they were not themselves medically qualified, their work considerably influenced the future of Medicine. They were Robert Grosseteste, Albertus Magnus, Vincent of Beauvois and Roger Bacon.

The unusually free and bold mind of Robert Grosseteste, Bishop of Lincoln from 1235-1253, brought the beginning of a new era to Oxford. After graduating there, and completing a period of postgraduate study in Paris, he returned to Oxford and became rector of a Franciscan Community (1224-1235). His importance arises from the influence which he exerted on several students, especially on a fellow Franciscan, Roger Bacon. A closely documented book by A. C. Crombie presents a strong case for regarding Grosseteste as the true fountain-head of the endeavours to unite logical coherence and a rational explanation of phenomena with experimental confirmations. Grosseteste aimed to define the conditions necessary for the validation of experimental results. He was the first medieval writer to wrestle with the methodological problems of verification and falsification, and his work was carried further by several successors in Oxford, such as Roger Bacon and William of Ockham. Grosseteste was specially interested in the question of the nature of light and he is believed to have stimulated in Bacon the latter's interest in optics.

A younger contemporary of Grosseteste in Germany, and one of Europe's most learned men of that time, was to become the dominant intellectual influence first in Paris and then in Cologne. Albert von Bollstadt (Albertus Magnus) was primarily a theologian and a philosopher, but he was also much interested in natural history. Educated in the Dominican communities of Germany and Paris, he returned to Germany and founded a university. Scattered through the writings of Albertus are a number of original observations and he encouraged the reader to validate facts by repeated observations. In addition to his theological and philosophical treatises, Albertus Magnus produced *De Vegetabilibus,* which is a summary guide to plants and minerals known to be useful in Medicine. His general influence on the universities and medical schools added greatly at the time to the general trend towards higher standards.

A third mind, in several ways similar to that of Albertus Magnus, especially in its capacity for immense industry, was that of Vincent de Beauvois. He too was a Dominican and, besides his theological writing, produced 'with the aid of several hundred authors' an encyclopaedia of all available knowledge, the *Speculum Majus* (Greater Mirror, or View). It is in three parts and the section entitled *Speculum Naturale* (Mirror of Nature) runs to 33 books. Several of these summarize the body of medical knowledge at that time. When printing was invented, an edition of the *Speculum Majus* was made in 1473-75. The main interest of this great project is the way in which the natural and applied sciences were beginning to take their place in the academic curriculum alongside more philosophical subjects.

Finally, in Roger Bacon the medieval universities received their most original, penetrating and far sighted man of genius — the 'Doctor Mirabilis'. He was, however, destined to be 'the first martyr in the cause of true research', for in the world of natural science and technology he became a catalyst undertaking a role similar to that which Luther was destined to play in the theological and ecclesiastical world. Bacon, however, was not permitted personally to carry his valuable insights and farsightedness into effect. On graduating at Oxford he entered the Franciscan Order and was transferred to a Franciscan monastery in Paris. Had not Pope Clement IV become his protector, the repression by the authorities of his Order would have inhibited further research. As it was, his brilliant promise was restricted and crushed following the death of Clement. Imprisoned for 14 years, he proved, on his release, to be a prematurely aged and broken man.

Roger Bacon was outstandingly brilliant whether viewed as theologian, philosopher, physician or natural scientist. His inventive genius and anticipation of the future were astonishing, and it is to the eternal shame of the ecclesiastical authorities responsible for restraining and suppressing such a mind that his abilities were not given every opportunity to work for the common good. Deeply influenced by Robert Grosseteste at Oxford, he gave rein to his early interests in mathematics, astronomy and chemistry, and more and more moved in the direction of experimental science. Early in his career he boldly asserted that if he could have his way he would burn all the books of Aristotle so as to end the current slavish dependence on him by all the philosophers and theologians. It would compel them to make their own observations and use their own minds. His familiar dictum was: 'Experiment is a firmer and more trustworthy basis of knowledge than argument.'

Roger Bacon was an advocate of the application of optics in ophthalmology. He knew of the refraction of light by a lens, the presence of the optic chiasma, and made a beginning of research into cerebral neurology. He is believed to have invented spectacles, using a convex lens to correct presbyopia. He also produced several practical monographs on matters of health, such as *Methods of Preventing the Onset of Senility.*

THREE INCENTIVES TO REFORM

The fall of Constantinople to the Turks in 1453, marking the end of the Byzantine Empire, brought new intellectual stimulus to the West. When the scholars fled they carried with them what they could of the classical manuscripts which had been preserved in the Byzantine libraries. They were welcomed by the enlightened rulers of Florence — Cosimo and Lorenzo de Medici. One result was the rebirth of classical scholarship and the recovery of much that had been forgotten. Interest also revived in Graeco-Roman knowledge of Medicine, especially as found in the Hippocratic writings.

The spread of the new learning received its second and most significant gain from the invention of printing. In 1456 Johannes Gutenberg presented Germany with the *Gutenberg Bible,* believed to have been Europe's first printed book, and in England Caxton's first production appeared some 20 years later. The further development of printing was to prove an invaluable and indispensable aid to the rapid circulation of all forms of learning.

From the point of view of the Christian religion, the third and epoch-making event came in 1517 when Martin Luther nailed his theses to the door of the castle church at Wittenburg. The Reformation had begun, though some years were to pass before it could achieve its full effects. All types of citizen were gradually drawn into the struggle. Among them were Christian physicians and surgeons who, mostly in secret but sometimes more openly, supported the reforming movements on intellectual and scientific, as well as religious, grounds. Several Christian medical practitioners were prominent among those who were working for intellectual liberty.

SIXTEENTH CENTURY LEADERS

The 16th century was dominated by four outstanding men, each of whom contributed to one of the growing departments of Medicine. They were (i) Andreas Vesalius, a Fleming from Brussels who led the way to accurate knowledge and illustration of human anatomy and put its teaching on to a new basis of fact; (ii) a German-speaking Swiss, 'Paracelsus,' who in his own strange manner was moving towards a new attitude in the practice of Medicine; (iii) a French Protestant, Ambroîse Paré, who introduced new techniques, compassion and hope into the practice of surgery; and (iv) an Italian, Girolamo Fracastoro, who put epidemiology and public health on to a new and scientific basis.

VESALIUS AND THE NEW ANATOMY

The university medical faculty at which the greatest progress in anatomy had so far been achieved was Paris. Several of the teachers there had been unobtrusively correcting some of the errors of Galen, whose dissecting of animals had led to a number of misleading views concerning the structure of some of the vital organs in the human body. For example, Jacques Dubois (Sylvius) seems to have been the first teacher of anatomy himself to dissect (that is personally and not through the proxy of a prosector) the whole of a human corpse. He had also been the first to inject dyes into the circulatory system so as to make the different vessels clearer for the dissector. It was, therefore, to Paris that Vesalius went for further study following his graduation in languages and mathematics at Louvain.

Another important influence which may have inspired Vesalius — that is, if it was known to him at the time — was the work of that versatile genius Leonardo da Vinci. Among the latter's many-sided interests was the structure of the human body, which awakened in him the constructive instincts of both artist and inventor. Starting with sketches of the muscles, Leonardo produced a series of superb drawings for an illustrated book on Anatomy prepared in conjunction with Marco della Torre of Pavia. The book, however, was left unfinished because of Marco's death. The drawings reveal original observation including, for example, the normal position of the fetus *in utero*. Leonardo also seems to have performed various experiments to determine the dynamics of the blood in circulation, to have injected wax into the cardiac ventricles, and to have demonstrated by use of models the functions of the opposing sets of muscles on a limb. He also described the atrioventricular bundle on the right side of the heart and the maxillary sinus in the skull.

Coming from a family in which there had been several prominent physicians, Vesalius now set himself the task of increasing accurate medical knowledge. Anatomy became his chief interest, and he applied himself to the dissection of the human body at considerable personal risk from action by the ecclesiastical authorities. For example, by some means he obtained possession of the bodies of several recently executed criminals and proceeded to dissect them secretly. At the early age of 22 he was invited to become Professor of Anatomy in the University of Padua. His epoch-making illustrated book of anatomy, *De Humani Corporis Fabrica* (Concerning the Structure of the Human Body), was published when he was only 29. In it he does not hesitate to differ from some of Galen's statements. Where the latter was writing from his dissection of animals, Vesalius was working from human subjects. Some of his drawings have never been surpassed.

Anatomists in other universities were not slow to take note of the significance of his work. Even so, enquiries by the Inquisition and the disapproval of his more 'orthodox' colleagues were not long in catching up with him. He therefore burnt the rest of his anatomical papers and left Padua to become court physician to the Emperor Charles V in Madrid. He had, however, already performed a valuable service to the future of Medicine.

The inclusion of Vesalius and some others in the series of pioneers raises again a problem which has already been touched upon. With the Renaissance and its impact on the intellectual outlook of Europe, there began to emerge a line of scientists who, while they had a Christian education and had been brought up in the national Church, were not always in later life clearly committed practising Christians themselves. The sparse available references to religious interests rarely make it clear how far a genius such as Vesalius was more than a humanist nominally identified with and practising the prevailing official religion. In 1563 he set out on a pilgrimage to Jerusalem and died on the return journey.

Vesalius' successor at Padua, Columbus of Cremona, who had been able to dissect as many as 14 bodies, courageously continued to correct Galen and even Vesalius from his own observations. It seems that he came very near to anticipating Harvey's work in the following century on the main circulation of the blood. He was certainly interested in the lesser circulation and described the heart's systole and diastole and related these to the pulsations of the arteries. It is surprising that he did not take the next step.

Another classical humanist — and one who clearly retained his definite Christian faith — was Thomas Linacre, physician to Henry VII and Henry VIII. Educated at Oxford and Padua, he returned to this country and practised in Oxford and taught Greek in the University. His expertise in the classical languages prompted him to complete more accurate Latin translations of Galen's works than those in common use. Linacre remained a Galenist and is best remembered for his founding of a Chair of Medicine at both Oxford and Cambridge which were, however, originally designed to further accurate exposition of the teachings of Hippocrates and Galen. By virtue of his position at Court, Linacre was also responsible for obtaining the King's patronage for the founding of the Royal College of Physicians in 1518.

THE NEW PHYSICIANS

One of the results of the arrival in Italy of the refugee scholars after the fall of Constantinople, bringing with them unknown or forgotten Greek texts (including some of the medical writings) was to give rise to what could be called a school of 'classical humanism'. The Professor of Medicine at Padua, Niccolo Leoniceno (or Leonicenus), who was a good linguist, speedily made excellent Latin translations of the medical texts, including the *Aphorisms* of Hippocrates. Leonicenus was bold enough not only to question the infallibility of Galen, but of Pliny in Natural History, by publishing a series of corrections to the latter's botanical and other biological writings. Indirectly the work of Leonicenus also increased the accuracy of the botanical descriptions in subsequent editions of the *Materia Medica*.

The physicians of the German-speaking lands were challenged early in the 16th century by a rugged pioneer of a very different mould. He was known as 'Paracelsus' but bore the perhaps appropriate full name of Philippus Aureolus Theophrastus Bombastus von Hohenheim. He was of Swiss nationality but was brought up in Austria at Villach in Carinthia. His father was the town doctor. He is believed to have studied medicine and qualified in Vienna and then to have taken a doctorate in Ferrara, but in the main he seems to have been self-educated. He certainly had a supreme contempt for those dependent only on book learning. Disillusioned with the contemporary curriculum and its slavish dependence on Galen, he soon made himself highly unpopular by saying so in no uncertain terms. On leaving university he travelled extensively all over Europe in search of empirical knowledge and observations in diagnosis and treatment. He then practised in Salzburg until he was appointed town doctor in Basel and professor of medicine in the university. Here his outspokenness and public burning of the books of Galen and others soon lost him this coveted post. He then began a life-long pilgrimage from place to place, staying and practising in one city until his unorthodoxy and ability to attract patients (the poor among them he treated free) united the opposition to his longer stay.

Opinions on the true nature and permanent influence of the work of Paracelsus have differed greatly. In the 16th century the misrepresentations of his enemies ensured him the reputation of a quack and imposter, but recent research, and especially the work of those who have gone more fully into his many hastily compiled writings, have presented a very different picture. Even so careful and knowledgeable an authority as William Osler could call him the 'Luther of Medicine'. Certainly Paracelsus did not help his own reputation either by his violent denunciation of Galen and Avicenna or in dogmatic assertions of his own

views. A basic ingredient in the trouble was his inherited and sturdy independence common to those reared in the mountains. As he exclaimed at
the end of his life: 'I have pleased no one, except the sick whom I cured.'

The total evidence suggests that Paracelsus was in fact a genius and that
several of his more important views were years before their time. He
certainly had an original and scientific mind. There are indications of the
vast amount of good which he did in each of the cities which kept him for
any length of time. There were several surprising cures of patients who
were regarded as incurable by local doctors. There is abundant evidence
of the widespread affection in which he was held by the masses. He
seemed to be the only doctor who understood them and would take
endless trouble to pursue a cure in each particular case. To the people he
was one of themselves who talked to them in their own language. Indeed,
one of his chief offences from the outset of his professorship at Basel was
that he insisted on lecturing to the students and writing in German.
Throughout his life he was commendably generous to the poor.

He regarded himself as a Christian in good standing, though he seems
to have been as 'empirical in some of his theological views as in his
scientific and medical outlook'. But he was always prepared to admit the
truth when he was wrong and to withdraw if given an adequate reason.
His life was all of a piece — a rugged, independently-minded genius who
ruthlessly pursued without fear or favour the good of any patient who put
his trust in him.

Paracelsus made a number of original observations and several additions to the pharmacopoeia. He was quick to note a connection between
cretinism and exophthalmic goitre in those districts where both were
prevalent. He also noted regional differences in the incidence of disease
and anticipated to a considerable extent what in recent times has come to
be called 'geographical pathology'. In his major book on surgery he
insisted on strict cleanliness in everything to do with surgical operations
and seems to have been the only person between de Mondeville in the
14th century and Semmelweiss and Lister in the 19th to have advocated
asepsis (in a rudimentary form). He introduced several extracts in alcohol
into the pharmacopoeia and he was one of the earliest physicians to
practise chemotherapy in its more modern forms. It has been objected
that there were elements of alchemy mixed with his elementary
chemistry. But, as has frequently been pointed out, much of what has
been dismissed as 'alchemy' were in those earlier times rudimentary
attempts to change basic chemical substances into other useful chemicals
— a process carried on today extensively in most scientific laboratories.

Surprisingly, Paracelsus was also a forerunner in what today would be called medical ethics. He was a strong advocate of the principle that the patient comes first, with such comments as: 'It is not the opinions which he holds, but the work he performs which constitutes a physician. This doctorship – this true understanding – is not conferred by emperors, or popes, or high schools, but is the gift of God.' Many a physician fails to find 'wisdom' and 'without this qualification all his learning will amount to little or nothing, so far as any benefit or usefulness to humanity is concerned. . . . A physician must seek for his knowledge and power within the divine spirit; if he seeks it in external things he will be a pseudo-medicus and an ignoramus. . . . He should exercise his art not for his own benefit, but for the sake of his patient.'

OTHER EMPIRICAL PHYSICIANS

Another physician who worked from bedside observations and from the elements of an empirical scientific approach was Guillaume de Baillou. He also wrestled with the menace of syphilis and endeavoured to solve the problem of 'the sweating sickness', though without success. But he clearly described relevant aspects of the pathology of the main organs of the body and the clinical differentiations of some of the infectious diseases such as whooping cough, scarlet fever, chicken pox, typhus and malaria.

The first of the regular physicians to make a firm break from the dominance of the Galenic-Arabic medical tradition was Pierre Brissot of Paris. He showed exemplary conviction and fortitude. It was in the practice of bloodletting that Brissot followed the Hippocratic method in bleeding, which was to take a large quantity at the outset from near the diseased site, whereas the Galenic-Arabic method was to take small quantities slowly in drops and at a distance from the affected part. During a severe epidemic of pneumonia in Paris in 1514, Brissot's approach was thought to be the more beneficial by far. His prestige in the city rose and his advocacy of the Hippocratic viewpoints and practice, together with his own careful observations, showed that he was feeling towards a new scientific outlook in Medicine.

RENAISSANCE SURGERY

As the surgeons and barber-surgeons were not so firmly controlled by the university medical faculties as were the physicians, a readiness to adopt an experimental approach tended to be stronger among them. The earliest innovations took place in central Europe among the army surgeons and, since firearms and artillery were becoming more and more used in war, the military surgeons began to show particular interest in the results of gunshot wounds. They also were beginning to write their case reports in the vernacular languages instead of Latin, and this process received a further stimulus when a successful French military surgeon, Ambroîse Paré, summarized in French for his fellow-countrymen the anatomical textbook of Vesalius, *De Fabrica*. With him came also the first clear signs of a radically progressive outlook in surgery.

Ambroîse Paré was the son of a cabinet maker and barber of Laval in Maine. His uncle was a barber-surgeon and Paré was first trained locally in that profession. Circumstances, however, permitted him to go to Paris and eventually he was fortunate to receive an appointment as an interne (house surgeon) at the Hôtel Dieu. He eventually qualified as a barber-surgeon, but since he had not been able to study at the university faculty (because of his lack of a Latin education) he had to be satisfied with only the humblest of qualifications from the independent college of surgeons of St. Côme.

It was only after nine years (1536-1545) of distinguished service in the army and his subsequently settling in Paris as court surgeon with access to the royal ear that (against strong opposition from the physicians of the university) he was invited by the Council of St. Côme to become a Fellow of that College.

During his military service Paré had treated the casualties sustained in numerous skirmishes and battles. He had acquired the reputation of being a most conservative surgeon and one of unusual practical industry in the care of his wounded patients. He had made efforts to perfect artificial limbs, including ingenious attempts to secure substitutes for hands. He became immensely popular among the soldiers. On leaving the army he was appointed to be one of the twelve royal surgeons and, later, the chief surgeon to Henry II, Francis II and Charles IX. This royal patronage was later to prove life-saving in his case, for there is no doubt that his sympathies were with the Huguenots. He is said to have been the 'only Protestant expressly exempted from the massacre on the eve of St. Bartholomew' and, on that occasion, he was ordered by Charles IX to stay the night in the royal apartments, where he was hidden in a wardrobe. He himself records a later unsuccessful attempt to poison him while he was on a journey to Lyon.

Paré's influence on the future of surgery arose less from the medical discoveries or the new techniques he introduced than from the fact that he effected a general change in the approach to the practice of surgery. His open-minded teaching, his unshakeable integrity and sympathetic caring attitude to the patient were unique in his day. In all his work he personified the virtues of unusual courage, common sense, practical industry and aptitude for research. He quietly sustained a resistance to medieval scholasticism and ecclesiastical repression. He met each professional crisis with a commendable honesty of mind and readiness to improvise.

How Paré came to abandon the usual and horrific use of the cautery in treating gunshot wounds has often been told but it bears repetition. The general view at that time was that such wounds were poisoned by gunpowder. Early in his war service, following the attack on the Château de Villare near Turin, his dressing station became overwhelmed by the numbers of wounded being brought in and the medical unit at last ran out of the boiling oil used for cauterizing. He therefore did the best he could to treat the rest of the wounded by an application of cold yolk of eggs and oil of roses in turpentine. Next day he found that all those in this second group had had a good night, had little or no pain, and that their wounds showed no inflammation. He there and then gave up using the cautery for military wounds. When later he was congratulated on the saving of a particularly severe case (in which he had personally dressed the wound several times) he replied in Old French, 'Je le pensyt, Dieu le guaryt' – I dressed it (the wound), God healed him. This became his constant attitude. He taught his generation respect for the patient and the spirit of true service. As he said, 'He who becomes a surgeon for the sake of knowledge will accomplish nothing,' and 'You will have to render an account not to the ancients, but to God for your humanity and skill.'

In thus calling attention to Paré's moral character and his inspiring example of service in practice, we must not overlook the fact that he possessed a high degree of scientific originality and that he introduced several important new techniques into surgery. In addition to the above mentioned methods for the treatment of wounds, he used ligatures in amputations (which were frequently necessary in military surgery) and to forestall haemorrhage in operations such as those for fistula-in-ano. He invented suitable trusses for hernias and a series of orthopaedic devices to replace lost limbs. Further he introduced podalic version (turning the baby into a better position) into the practice of obstetrics, and constructed specially shaped bottles for the artificial feeding of invalids. He was the first to note fully the sequelae to fractures of the femur, to recognize the results of certain renal conditions and of an enlarged prostate, and to suggest that many aneurysms were the result of the action of syphilis on the wall of an artery. He corrected hare-lip by the use of a figure-of-eight suture and even ventured into the making of artificial eyes. He several times managed successfully to implant a tooth, obtained from *paid* donors!

Paré has good claim to be regarded as one of the chief liberators of surgery from long-established erroneous ideas. An indication of the spirit in which he carried out his professional service is given in his little book advocating the care with which a surgeon should write up any surgical report such as, for example, the pathological conditions found at a post-mortem examination. 'It is very expedient that a Chirurgion be of an honest mind, that he may always have before his eyes a careful regard of true piety, that is to say, the fear of God and faith in Christ, and love towards his neighbours with hope of life everlasting, lest that he being carried away by favour, or corrupted with money or rewards, should affirm or testify those wounds to be small that are great, and those great that are small; for the report of a wound is received of the Chirurgion according to the Civil Law.'

FRACASTORO AND THE NEW PUBLIC HEALTH

Several other branches of Medicine showed signs of progress in the 16th century and there are good reasons why the physician Girolamo Fracastoro should be regarded as 'the father of modern pathology'. He was another classical humanist who, as Sigerist comments, was 'on good terms with the Church'. He was one of those versatile geniuses who were equally at home in medicine, pathology, physics, geology and astronomy. In physics he was the first to recognize and discuss the earth's magnetic poles and he was one of the first in geology to suggest a modern view concerning the origin of fossil beds. Fracastoro enrolled in Padua as a student in 1501, the same year as Copernicus entered the university.

His medical reputation mainly rests on a long poem, *De Contagione et Contagiosis morbis* (Concerning Contagion and Contagious Disease), 1546. In this he shows a clear grasp of the origin and spread of epidemic diseases. He suggests that they are conveyed by little seeds or particles, and he classifies them as follows: (i) those spread by personal contacts, such as leprosy, scabies and respiratory tuberculosis; (ii) those transferred by indirect contact, e.g. by utensils and bedclothes as in some of the fevers; and (iii) those which seem to traverse distances, e.g. smallpox. He also recognized that the 'seeds' of infectious diseases can multiply very quickly. In several of his findings Fracastoro came very close to modern concepts of infectious disease. His work was supplemented by that of Guillaume de Baillou (p. 52) who revived the view put forward by Hippocrates that particular seasons of the year were more favourable to the spread of certain diseases and that their virulence also varied with the climate. Thomas Sydenham in 1666 was to take further this concept of 'epidemic constitutions'.

To look back over the years from the early Church through the centuries dominated by the medieval Church until the Reformation is to be impressed by the frequent disparity between the organized institutions in both Church and Medicine and the individual. On the institutional side the authorities were frequently in error, sometimes corrupt, and in general tended to be jealous and repressive of genius. Perhaps this was inevitable in view of human nature's self-centredness and ambitions, though the Church did not quite forget the example of its Founder and the command to heal the sick. It was, however, in marked contrast with the nobility of spirit in which over those centuries the long line of devoted individual practitioners and members of the nursing sisterhoods served the interests of the sick and advanced the efficiency of the profession.

CHAPTER 5

THE RISE OF MODERN SCIENCE

IN Western Europe by the opening of the 17th century the 'new learning' had had time to make itself effectively felt in most spheres of national life. Several factors favoured its fuller application to the public's needs as well as those of the learned professions. Scientists began to lecture and write in the vernacular instead of Latin. The timely invention of printing had been furthered by technical advances in type-making, paper manufacturing and binding. This enabled larger editions of books to be undertaken and new trade routes provided them with an international circulation.

During this century in the main cities and some of the universities scientific societies were started. Some of these eventually became fertile centres of basic research. Exchanges of correspondence and the transactions reporting their findings led to an increasing co-operation, sometimes at international levels. Wealthier members and some of the societies themselves began to build up specialist libraries. Several groups also began to collect geological and biological specimens forming the first natural history museums. The feature which was common to all these societies was their devotion to the observations of 'experimental philosophy' with its inductive method. Their memberships often contained a high proportion of graduates with medical qualifications. One such group was the Royal Society in London. Not, however, until the following century did doctors begin to have similar, but exclusively medical, societies.

CHRISTIAN SUPPORT

In all these developments active Christians played a considerable, sometimes a central, part. The economy of some of the more prosperous printing and publishing houses depended substantially on Christian interests, for example in printing the growing number of translations of the Bible into the vernaculars, together with new Prayer Books and the writings of the Reformers and other theologians. The majority of the ablest ministers in the reformed Churches were sympathetic to the new scientific outlook. Also, the 'experimental philosophy' was specially welcomed in their medical thinking by doctors who, like Sydenham, were themselves Puritans or were sympathetic to Puritanism.

It is to be regretted that several standard histories of Medicine have continued to repeat misrepresentations of the views of Calvin and several others of the chief reformers. These views have been taken over from writers who were unsympathetic to the Reformation and the Puritans, so that less than justice has been done to some of the early benefactors of modern science. When we examine the evidence carefully, it is clear that the scientific activities of the infant Royal Society arose from a decidedly Christian matrix, although its members were drawn from different backgrounds in that some had been Royalists and others Parliamentarians during the Civil War.

In recent years two impressive studies have been published which have sought to correct the historical perspective. Each comes from an historian well versed in this field. The Croall Lectures of 1969 in the University of Edinburgh were presented by R. Hooykaas, Professor of the History of Science in the University of Utrecht. His thesis was 'Religion and the Rise of Science', and this was published in a stimulating small volume in 1972. In 1975 came Charles Webster's truly monumental study The Great Instauration: Science, Medicine and Reform, 1626-1660. The following paragraphs summarize some of the relevant facts from these sources.

FRANCIS BACON

The intellectual pedigree of the thinking which became characteristic of the early members of the Royal Society goes back to Francis Bacon who was a devout member of the Church of England and in his writing was aiming to organize education and scientific research on a Christian basis. While Bacon himself was to contribute little original to the sum of scientific knowledge, he proved to be the eloquent herald of 'experimental philosophy' and the major influence on the next generation of English scientists.

In The Advancement of Learning, the Novum Organum and the New Atlantis Bacon urged the need for a Great Design covering the national organization, or reorganization, of education, and research in the arts, sciences and technologies. His plan included the founding of an international postgraduate college which would be controlled by the wisest and ablest living scholars. Fundamentally, he was calling for the end of the agelong domination of Aristotle and the classical philosophers (by whom Nature had been virtually worshipped as divine) and the substitution of a thoroughly Christian view of life and the world.

Bacon's favourite illustration of the basic need was to speak of God as having given mankind two books, (i) the theological revelation in Holy Scripture, to which man can only respond in faith and trust; and (ii) the revelation of his created works, into the phenomena of which he is free (and indeed has been invited) to search. In Bacon's view man could scarcely go too fully and deeply into either book, but the different attitude in which each was to be approached was of crucial importance. In the case of the second book he proposed that the correct approach was by the means of the inductive method of 'the experimental philosophy'.

Bacon did not believe, or suggest, that Book I was in error or in any conflict with Book II, but their purpose and the attitude in which they were to be received were different. Like Calvin and some of the leading reformed theologians, he believed that in Book I God had condescended, in deference to man's intellectual limitations, to speak of scientific things in the popular language of everyday common sense, whereas in reading Book II the 'experimental philosopher' is free to assemble his observations, make his tests and adapt his terminology in keeping with the empirical findings. This to many of the Puritans was their *philosophia libera,* liberating them intellectually from the misunderstandings and strait-jacket of the classical and medieval authorities.

As Hooykaas comments, 'According to Bacon there are two sources of theological error: that of ignoring the *will* of God, revealed in Scripture, and that of ignoring the *power* of God, revealed or made visible in His creatures.' Bacon even held that Christ, when saying, 'You err, not knowing the Scriptures, nor the power of God,' was referring to the two books, the Scriptures and the creatures.

In his exhaustive study Webster traces the optimism of those with Puritan sympathies who believed that the establishment of the Commonwealth had ushered in the promised golden age of the millennium (Rev. 20). Taking Bacon's *Instauratio Magna* (the Great Design) as their model, they began to take steps to organize the activities of education and research around it. In keeping with Bacon's project of a Universal College, they also planned a higher 'intellectual command', centred in their prototype of a postgraduate research college. Their hopes were doomed to disappointment. Civil wars and their aftermaths are not the best of circumstances in which to attempt major research. From the point of view of Medicine, however, it is striking to read of a growing interest in the subject. During the last ten years of the Commonwealth (1650-1660) roughly *ten* times the number of new books on Medicine were published (and only *three* times the number in the important subjects of mathematics and agriculture) as compared with the first ten years of the 17th century (1600-1610).

THE ROYAL SOCIETY

While the Royal Society was not fully constituted until 1660, and did not receive its royal charter from Charles II until 1663, there had already been several groups of intellectuals who had been meeting for scientific purposes. Several of their members were later to become the foundation members of the Royal Society. The earliest of these circles met around the year 1645 and consisted of mathematicians, scientists and medicals. Their earliest meetings were at their favourite inns, but later they assembled after the public lectures at Gresham's College and so came to be known as the Gresham Group. These 'divers worthy persons, inquisitive into natural philosophy, and particularly what was called the New Philosophy or Experimental Philosophy' met weekly to pursue 'philosophical inquiries'. Because of the diversity of their other interests, religious affiliations and political loyalties, they made a rule that 'Matters of theology and State affairs' should be excluded from their discussions.

In 1646, through the initiative of Robert Boyle, son of the Earl of Cork, a study group of Irishmen (who were mostly graduates from Trinity College, Dublin) began to meet in the house of his sister, Lady Ranelagh. Boyle refers to it as their Invisible College, because it had no buildings of its own and worked only by its meetings and correspondence. By an error of its historians this title has been applied to the Royal Society and appears in its histories. The College aimed to pursue practical subjects which 'have a tendency to use', and the members were pledged to research and social action.

At the close of the Civil War, about 1648-49, some of the members of the Gresham Group were given posts in Oxford. For example, John Wilkins (Cromwell's brother-in-law) became Warden of Wadham College and a physician, William Petty (later Cromwell's personal physician in Ireland), a fellow and Vice-Principal of Wadham College. Robert Boyle also took lodgings in Oxford for several years. Through the initiative of the hospitable Wilkins, who invited interested persons to his lodgings in Wadham, a new circle of experimenters grew up to become known as the Philosophical Club, later the Experimental Philosophy Club. Eventually, at the Restoration, when a number of the leading men removed to London, there was a united meeting in 1660 between these Oxford men and those of the Gresham Group who had remained in London. They met to discuss the founding of a college to promote 'Physico-Mathematical Experimental Philosophy'. This united body later became the Royal Society.

Both Hooykaas and Bennett have demonstrated that in both the memberships and initiatives of these early groups, and also in the resulting Royal Society, there was a high proportion of Puritans and those who sympathized with them. Hooykaas quotes the American sociologist, Professor R. K. Martin, who wrote in 1938: 'Among the group of ten scientists who during the Commonwealth formed the nucleus of the body which was to become the Royal Society, seven were strongly Puritan. Sixty-two per cent of the members in 1663 were clearly Puritan by origin, a percentage that is the more striking because the Puritans constituted a minority of the population.' In addition to those who were of Puritan outlook, there were others best described as devout Anglicans on the model of Charles I's physician William Harvey. Though not himself a member of the groups described, Harvey had shown himself fully in sympathy with their aims and with the experimental philosophy. During his residence with the King in Oxford, and his brief administration as Warden of Merton College, Harvey had gathered around him a group of younger men to carry further his researches into embryology. Several of these men from Oxford later became members of the Royal Society.

The importance to our theme of the history of this momentous period is that the great majority of the early pioneer scientists, intent on applying the experimental inductive method in researches, were devout Christians. Their motivation, the dynamic in their commendable industry and in their intellectual endeavours were essentially Christian. Some of the more prominent among the physicians of this period deserve further attention.

WILLIAM HARVEY

A key date in history was 1628, which saw the publication of Harvey's *De Motu Cordis* (Concerning the Heart's Movements), in which he described his experiments demonstrating the nature of the circulation of the blood.

Several physicians in earlier times had come close to a solution of the problem, but now there was clear experimental demonstration of the phenomenon, a fact that did much to confirm the value of the experimental approach. Harvey had been engaged on other work of medical value but on the outbreak of the Civil War he, as the royal physician, accompanied Charles I on his campaigns and when the Court settled in Oxford in 1640, was in residence there for several years. During the next year Harvey's lodgings in Whitehall were pillaged and most of his books and papers containing research notes, observations and recordings were lost. At the age of 60 he was in no mood for repeating the work or replacing these documents. But, as described above, when appointed Warden of Merton College he encouraged the group of younger workers in several new avenues of research.

In his biography of Harvey Geoffrey Keynes writes: 'Harvey was reticent concerning his religious beliefs. But passages in *De Generatione Animalium* (1651), edited and published by George Ent, give evidence of a profound awareness of Divine Providence supervising human life and maintaining the laws of nature.' His intimate friend Charles Scarburgh commented that Harvey always cherished 'that philosophy which had reverence for Divine authority and uprightness of character so that he might regulate his life with integrity'.

ROBERT BOYLE

Because of his consistent interest in experimental science and his ability to finance a good deal of their work, Robert Boyle became a central figure in the Invisible College, the Gresham Group, the Oxford Experimental Philosophy Club and in the first years of the Royal Society. In boyhood he had had deep spiritual convictions and showed a prodigious capacity for memorizing the Scriptures. In his teens he became proficient in Greek and Latin and, for good measure, added Hebrew, Chaldean and Syriac. When, later, he had received the Oxford M.D. he spent a good deal of time on medical research. He preferred not to practise but to continue as an experimental scientist.

His main interests and researches into the behaviour of gases are well known and immortalized in Boyle's Law. But throughout his life his scientific interests were very wide. He experimented on animals in a vacuum and showed that air was necessary both to life and combustion. The full list of the work done in his laboratories is surprising. In the sphere of Medicine he investigated a series of possible therapeutic measures, studied such phenomena as the work of Valentine Greatraks (the Irish hypnotist) and completed fundamental work on the lungs, renal structures and nervous systems, including the investigation of the reflexes. He published *Humane Blood,* the first English study of blood biochemistry, and also *Porosity of Bodies,* which was a beginning of physiological studies into the importance of osmotic pressures.

In almost every way Boyle is the embodiment of the ideal Christian 'experimental philosopher'. For to him there was no tension between a deep practical faith and wholehearted devotion to empirical research in all branches of science. He made this clear throughout his writings by such remarks as 'Greatness of mind is promoted by Christianity' and his reminder 'of the high veneration which man's intellect owes to God peculiarly for His wisdom and power'. Speaking of medical practice he claimed 'that by being addicted to experimental philosophy, a man is rather assisted than indisposed to be a good clinician'.

His Christian charity was far-reaching and illustrated by such imaginative major undertakings as paying for the translation and publication of the first Gaelic Bible and the presentation of copies to each of the local Churches in Ireland and Scotland. He paid for translations of the Bible into Turkish, Arabic, Malayan and Indian (of North America). He also endowed the Boyle lectures in defence of the Christian Faith to be given in Lincoln's Inn Chapel. Among his collected works are several treatises on theological subjects.

BOYLE'S TRAINEES AND OTHERS

By employing them as assistants in his own experiments and subsidizing them for their own original work, Boyle was responsible for encouraging a number of younger scientific writers. His chief assistant, Robert Hooke, son of the curate of Freshwater, Isle of Wight, went on to demonstrate the aerating function of the lungs. He proved to be scientifically very versatile, becoming an active microscopist and being the first to use the word 'cell' for the microstructures of plants and animals.

Another of Boyle's assistants, Richard Lower, noted that exposure to air made blood corpuscles turn red. Wondering whether this was what happened in the lungs, he repeated Hooke's experiments and also noticed that the blood of an animal turned dark when artificial respiration was stopped. He was one of the earliest to experiment with blood transfusion in animals. He also noticed that 'a running nose in a cold' was due to inflammation of the mucous membranes and not to 'purging of the brain' as was commonly thought at the time.

Thomas Willis became Professor of Natural Philosophy at Oxford. He is known to have been of one mind with many devout Christians, including Harvey and Robert Boyle's group. Curiously, however, he still held to some of the outmoded theories of Galen on medical practice rather than, as one would have expected, the new experimental theories. But he became interested in the gases produced by fermentation, identified sugar in the urine of diabetic patients, and is best remembered for his atlas of the brain and especially for the arterial 'circle of Willis'. The illustrations for his book *Cerebri Anatome* (1664) were mostly drawn for him by that many-sided genius, the architect Christopher Wren. Willis was also an observant clinician. It was he who first described myasthenia gravis, epidemic typhoid (in *De Febribus*) and puerperal fever, which he also named. Of immediate practical aid to colleagues was his publication in 1674 of a summary of the *Materia Medica.*

During that period of turmoil and reconstruction, and after the Restoration, there were numbers of prominent medical practitioners among both the Royalist and Puritan ranks who revealed strong Christian motivation for their work. When the Clarendon Code of 1662 closed Oxford and Cambridge to them, the Nonconformists developed a number of advanced educational institutions which became known as the Dissenting Academies. From them were destined to come medical leaders such as Thomas Percival, and scientists such as Joseph Priestley and John Dalton.

TWO OUTSTANDING PHYSICIANS

The best day-to-day practice of 17th century physicians is well illustrated by the lives of two eminent practitioners, Thomas Browne of Norwich and Thomas Sydenham of London.

Thomas Browne practised in the city of Norwich for 46 years and, having been chosen as its most worthy resident, was knighted by Charles I in gratitude for citizens' support during the Civil War. He was a most conscientious practitioner and one of the first to write on the problems of medical ethics. His best known book, *Religio Medici,* is still being published, and for over 300 years it has exercised a wide and salutary influence. The manuscript is believed to have been started early in his career when he was still an apprentice to a practitioner near Oxford, and to have been finished during his earliest years in practice in Norwich.

Throughout his life Thomas Browne continued to reflect on the responsibility of a doctor and the ethics of the medical profession. He returns to the subject again and again. 'I am a medical man,' he says, 'and this is my religion. I am a physician, and this is my faith and my morals, and my whole true and proper life. The scandal of my profession, the natural course of my studies, and the indifference of my behaviour and discourse in matters of religion, might persuade the world that I had no religion at all. And yet, in despite of all that, I dare, without usurpation, to assume the honourable style of a Christian.'

In some notes in his private papers (not intended for publication, but for his son) he wrote his resolve: 'To be sure that no day pass without calling upon God in a solemn, fervent prayer, seven times within the compass thereof. . . . To pray in all places where privacy inviteth: in any house, highway, or street: and to know no street or passage in this city which may not witness that I have not forgot God and my Saviour in it. . . . To take occasion of praying upon the sight of any church which I see or pass as I ride about. . . . Upon sight of beautiful persons, to bless God for His creatures and to pray for the beauty of their souls. . . . Upon sight of deformed persons, to pray Him to send them inward graces, and to enrich their souls, and give them the beauty of the resurrection.'

Browne was indeed a devout Christian who, even in those days when searching questions were already being raised, sought to reconcile science and religion. When not on duty his recreation was to explore the natural history of the Eastern counties.

Thomas Sydenham has the reputation of being one of the outstanding pioneers of clinical medicine. He came of a Puritan and Parliamentary family, and his father and four brothers were all in Cromwell's army. While at Oxford he was friendly with Robert Boyle and John Locke the philosopher. He became known as the 'English Hippocrates' because of his careful bedside observations and his descriptions of the course taken by various diseases. His clinical descriptions were much admired by the celebrated Dutch physician Herman Boerhaave, Professor of Medicine in Leyden University and himself a distinguished clinician, who paid tribute to Sydenham's influence when he (Boerhaave) introduced bedside teaching into the Continental medical schools. Sydenham was much opposed to the complicated prescriptions (and their often bizarre contents) given by the physicians of the day, and was very conservative in his treatment of all patients. His contributions to medical teaching include classical descriptions of gout and chorea, and the differences between a number of the common infectious diseases.

Sydenham was a man of deep piety and some of his recorded prayers are still appropriate to current medical practice. In *Medical Observations concerning the History and Cure of Acute Diseases*, published in 1668, Sydenham wrote: 'Whoever takes up Medicine should seriously consider that he must one day render to the Supreme Judge an account of the lives of those sick men who have been entrusted to his care. Secondly, that such skill and science as, by the blessing of Almighty God, he has attained, are to be specially directed towards the honour of his Maker, and the welfare of his fellow-creatures: since it is a base thing for the great gifts of heaven to become the servants of avarice and ambition. Thirdly he must remember that it is no mean or ignoble animal that he deals with. We may ascertain the worth of the human race, since for its sake God's only begotten Son became man, and thereby ennobled the nature that He took upon Him.'

'Lastly, he (the doctor) must remember that he himself has no exemption from the common lot, but that he is bound by the same laws of mortality and liable to the same ailments and afflictions with his fellows. For these and like reasons let him strive to render aid to the distressed with the greater care, with the kindlier spirit, and with the stronger fellow feeling.'

SURGERY AND TROPICAL MEDICINE

The leading military surgeon in England at this time was Richard Wiseman, an active member of St. Paul's Church, Covent Garden. He was in many ways as outstanding in surgery as Sydenham was in medicine, and his *Several Chirurgical Treaties* (1672) circulated as the standard book of surgery for many years. He was a Royalist and became surgeon to Charles I and Charles II. Wiseman made a special study of gunshot wounds and practised amputation when there were gunshot wounds of the joints. He gave a classic description of the white swellings accompanying tuberculous infection of the joints.

Peter Lowe was a prominent surgeon in Glasgow and a medical reformer. He aimed to bring together practitioners from the four main fields: the apothecaries, the barber-surgeons, the surgeons and the physicians. In the event he succeeded and became a founder member of the (united) Faculty of Physicians and Surgeons in Glasgow. Among his non-medical writings are found a commentary on Ecclesiastes, in the last chapter of which he pays special attention to the description of old age and death.

Another surgeon, John Woodall, was responsible for one of the most influential books on surgery at this period, *The Surgions Mate* (1617). It is partly a surgeon's *vade mecum,* combined with an apprentice's guide to learning and good conduct. Woodall was anxious to make it quite clear where the surgeon's duty and responsibility lay. 'The office and duty of the Surgeon's mate may, in my opinion, well be divided into three parts, whereof the first concerns his duty to God, who sees not as men see, who is a searcher of the hearts. . . . St. Paul advises servants to obey froward masters, so I advise Surgeon's mates to do the like to froward surgeons. . . . The first errors some young surgeons are possessed with, from which infinite others grow, is the want of the service of God, the example whereof to their mates is very infectious.'

In practical treatment he shows some progress in those times, for example Woodall was aware of the value of 'the juice of lemons, a good preservative' in relation to scurvy. He also wrote, 'the use of juice of lemons is a precious medicine and well tried'.

The first book in English on medicine in the tropics was *A Discourse on the State of Health in the Island of Jamaica* by Thomas Trapham. During the Civil War he had been a surgeon with the Parliamentary forces and 'body-surgeon' to Cromwell. After the Restoration he settled at Abingdon which was at that time a centre for nonconformity.

PROTESTANT REFUGEES AND EVICTED MINISTERS

During this century the Christian forces in this country were strengthened by a number of doctors who were among the Protestant refugees escaping to the countries bordering on France. They formed a welcome addition to those working for higher professional standards. An outstanding example was Gideon Delaune. He was the son of a French Protestant minister who had studied medicine in Paris and Montpellier and came to England to escape the religious persecution. Delaune re-qualified in London as an apothecary and was attached to the entourage of Queen Anne of Denmark at the court of James I. He was largely instrumental in securing the separation of the apothecaries from the Grocers' Company and he became Master of the Company of Apothecaries in 1637. It was largely through his generous donations that the Company flourished and the Apothecaries Hall was acquired.

In 1662, under the Clarendon Code following the Restoration of

Charles II, there was a second ejection, this time of Puritan ministers from the Church of England. Nearly 2000 could not conscientiously comply with the new formularies and, as they were forbidden to teach, a number turned to the study of Medicine and entered the medical profession. Among them was Richard Morton. After his ejection in 1662 he received an Oxford M.D. in 1670 and became a fellow of the Royal College of Physicians in 1679. Later he was physician to the King. He published two significant books which were regarded as the best on the subjects for some years. In *Phthisiologia* he describes at length tuberculosis and its symptoms and signs. He had studied the process of the formation of tubercles in the lung and observed that there was often spontaneous healing. In *Pyretologia* he discussed the infectious fevers, especially scarlet fever (which, however, he did not distinguish from measles).

ON THE CONTINENT

Jan Swammerdam, the Dutch microscopist and physician was a devout Christian. He is noted for his discovery of the valves of lymph vessels and the identification of red blood cells. He also showed that the lungs of an infant would float only if the child had breathed. Thomas Bartholin, a Danish anatomist, described the greater vestibular gland and was one of the first to recognize the significance of the lymphatic system. He was among those doctors who have written books which discuss the diseases of the Bible.

Another pioneer in anatomy was Niels Stensen (Steno) of Denmark, who became interested in the ductless glands. He discovered the duct from the parotid gland which is named after him. In his *Observationes Anatomicae* he showed that other secretory glands have similar ducts, for example the lacrimal apparatus of the eye. Among other anatomical-physiological work he demonstrated the action of the fibrils of muscles in muscle contraction. Disappointed at not being appointed to the chair of anatomy in Copenhagen, he went to Italy, joined the Roman Catholic Church, and rose to the rank of bishop.

Jacob Benignus Winslow was of Danish birth but lived most of his life in Paris where he became well known as an anatomist, but one with a difference. For while working as a highly respected general practitioner, he studied the organs of the body *in situ,* being at the same time equally interested in their physiological functions and interrelationships. For example, he was the first to describe the foramen of Winslow in the abdomen and he did much to systematize the existing knowledge of the origins, insertions and functioning of the different muscles. Brought up in a Lutheran family in Denmark, he found the formal barrenness of the Danish Church of the time not to his taste and, like Steno, he later became a Roman Catholic.

It was the German physician G. E. Stahl who formulated the erroneous phlogiston theory of combustion, an explanation which was reversed by Lavoisier 100 years later. However, he was responsible for one of the salutary shifts of thinking and attitudes in Medicine. Stahl belonged to the Pietist movement. He is important because he exerted a strong influence in opposing the crude materialistic views of the human being which were coming to the fore at that time. He taught that the body was not governed simply by natural materialistic laws, but by a sensitive soul. The physician's personal and clinical attitude to the patient should be controlled by that fact. In his *De Animi Morbis* (on Mental Diseases) Stahl was the first to emphasize that certain mental states are of physical origin, while others are functional. He was also among the first writers to call attention to the influence of the body on the mind and of the mind on the body.

One of the most influential observers and experimenters on the Continent was Jan Baptista van Helmont. Born in Brussels, he attended the University of Louvain and was for a time a friar. Then, after a grand tour of Europe, he married a wealthy heiress and settled on her estate in Vilvarden to concentrate on his studies of Chemistry as applied to Medicine. His outlook represents the growing tension between sceptism and faith which was affecting many in this period. Here was a deeply religious man who, at the same time, wished creatively to follow the new avenues which were being opened up by experimental science. Influenced by the writings of Paracelsus, he resolved to apply himself to the study of the natural sciences with a view to their use in therapeutics. While, in the event, his views became something of an ill-assorted mixture of 'idealistic-spiritualistic and empirical-scientific' elements, yet he made several advances. For example, he discovered carbon dioxide and introduced the word 'gas'. His importance as a pioneer is that he took the first steps towards biochemistry, and he may be considered as the first chemical physiologist.

The somewhat complicated and mystical thought of Paracelsus and van Helmont was given a clearer and more practical turn by Francois de la Boë (or Sylvius) who was primarily an anatomist. Born in Germany of a French Huguenot family, he attended German and Dutch universities and eventually became Professor of Medicine at Leyden. Especially through such pupils as Willis in England, de Graaf and Swammerdam in Holland and Stensen in Denmark, his influence was strong in emphasizing the importance of anatomy to medicine and in popularizing Harvey's work on the circulation. His name is perpetuated in the fissure of Sylvius in the brain. In clinical medicine he was a leading teacher in the art of clinical observation and the empirical application of new treatment, including chemical substances. He gave much attention to the reactions of acids, alkalis and fermentation, especially those concerned with digestion. He suggested that digestion was a form of fermentation and outlined the functions of saliva and the pancreatic excretion. He also forecast later findings in physiology regarding the functions of the ductless glands. He was thus another of the pioneer chemical physiologists.

THE PLAGUE DOCTORS

An interesting sidelight on the work of general practitioners in London in the 17th century is given in Bell's *The Great Plague of London.* When the richer citizens moved out of the city from the plague and made for the outer suburbs and country, most of the fashionable physicians and surgeons moved out with them, as did those in all the professions. This reduced still more the already inadequate provision of medical care for the lower ranks of the populace. Some of the London practitioners, however, did not move out and it appears that the majority of those who remained were deeply religious men with a strong sense of public duty. For example, John Allin, who was one of the clergy ejected in 1662 and who took up Medicine, was among those who remained. Because of his nonconformist religious views he had been unable to obtain a medical licence and was practising without one, but there were few or none of the leaders of the profession to question the good he was doing. His letters 'reveal the thoughts and emotions of an intelligent observer confined to the City, whilst all lay sick and dying of the Great Plague'. Of these brave 'plague doctors' most prominent and widely respected was Nathaniel Hodges, son of the Vicar of Kensington, who is said later to have become a Baptist. He remained in London and resolutely responded to all who sought his aid. In his book *Loimologia* (Treatise on the Pestilence) he provides a vivid and classical account of the symptoms, signs and course of the plague. It is good to read that his work was at length recognized by his election to a Fellowship of the Royal College of Physicians in 1672 and his being invited to give the Harveian Oration in 1683.

CHAPTER 6

SOME PROMINENT EIGHTEENTH CENTURY PRACTITIONERS

NOT until the 18th Century were the medical professions of Europe beginning to be better regulated by appropriate authorities. Even then much was left to be desired, although in the more progressive countries the colleges and guilds of physicians and surgeons were beginning to improve the required standards of training. A few steps were also being taken in medical ethics and medical 'etiquette' to provide better relations and cooperation between practitioners. It was not, however, until the mid-19th century that the state entered the field and prescribed standards of teaching and required official registration of those who were qualified to practise.

It was an age of outstanding personalities and among them were a number of able medical practitioners, some of whom began to develop what were to become specialist branches of a greatly enlarged field of Medicine. Among these were not a few devout Christians.

The 17th and 18th centuries might also be called the age of the 'great collectors' for many wealthy men brought together large collections of books, natural history specimens, antiquities, medals, coins and much else. A noteworthy example was Sir Hans Sloane, a prominent London physician, whose collection after his death formed the original holdings of the British Museum. Sloane was born in Ulster of Scottish Presbyterian stock, though when in London he became a member and benefactor of Chelsea Parish Church. He later bought the Manor of Chelsea and rebuilt the mansion to house his collections.

Sloane was an able botanist and succeeded Sir Isaac Newton as President of the Royal Society. During 15 months in Jamaica he studied the flora of the island and brought home with him many Caribbean plants. Becoming interested in the Chelsea Physic Garden in 1722 he purchased it and made it over to the impoverished Society of Apothecaries for a nominal rent 'to enable the society to support the charge thereof; for the manifestation of the power, wisdom and glory of God in the works of Creation'. He became a President, and a generous benefactor, of the Royal College of Physicians. While he himself made no

71

outstanding contribution to medical science, as a pupil of Sydenham, and court physician to more than one monarch, he was a much sought after practitioner and benefactor to Medicine. He was an advocate of the use of Peruvian bark (quinine) and of the early practice of inoculation, which led to vaccination.

Another of the best known London physicians at the time was Richard Mead who was the son of a clergyman who was ejected from his church in Stepney because of his refusal to conform under the Acts of Charles II. Mead received his education from nonconformist colleges and later studied Medicine at Leyden and Padua. He returned to Stepney to practise, but in 1726 moved to a house in Great Ormond Street, on the site of which now stands the well known Children's Hospital. In his practice he is said to have been without a rival and his average income over several years was enormous, considering the value of money at that time. It is good to be able to add that 'his charity and his hospitality were unbounded'. For example, a fellow London practitioner, Friend, was committed to the Tower for political reasons. Mead took over his practice and used his influence to obtain Friend's release. He subsequently handed over to him several thousand pounds which represented the fees he had collected from Friend's patients during his internment.

Fears were aroused in Britain by an outbreak of plague at Marseilles in 1720, and Mead was invited by a secretary of state to write a short volume on its prevention and treatment. This appeared as *Treatise concerning Pestilential Contagion*. Mead, however, reflected the contemporary views on the disease and, had the plague again struck this country, the practices he recommended would have done little to check it. Mead collected one of the best libraries in Britain and also a large museum, which became a centre for visitors. He also worked to encourage progress in research.

In 1751 he published the most important of his works, *Monita et Praecepta Medica* (Medical Precepts and Cautions). 'Compared with similar productions of its epoch, this book stands high on the ground of judgement and taste; it is generally free from the superstitious poly-pharmacy which defaces many of its contemporaries.' Mead was one of those physicians who attempted to bridge the gulf that had arisen between the physician and the apothecary by making his experience available to the latter. His contemporary, Samuel Johnson, wrote of him that he lived more in the broad sunshine of life than almost any man. After his retirement he wrote *Medica Sacra,* a commentary on the diseases mentioned in Scripture. He says: 'I frequently read the Holy Scriptures as becomes a Christian, and next to those things which regard eternal life and the doctrine of mortality, I usually give particular attention to the histories of diseases and various ailments therein recorded, comparing those with what I have learned either from medical authors or my own experience.'

A prominent surgeon, Thomas Chevalier, was of Huguenot extraction and a deacon of Keppel Street Baptist Church. He studied under Matthew Baillie, nephew of the Hunters, and became a distinguished member of the London Corporation of Surgeons. Appointed surgeon to the Westminster Dispensary, he produced a volume on gunshot wounds in 1804, and was given the Chair of Anatomy and Surgery at the College of Surgeons. He was also appointed surgeon to the Prince of Wales. In his own day he was esteemed not only as a surgeon and anatomist but as a linguist and theologian. He translated Bousset's *Universal History* and Pascal's *Pensées,* and he also wrote the preface to Bagster's Polyglot Bible.

Edward Hulse was one of the group of clergymen who, ejected from their pulpits by the Act of Settlement of 1662, took up medicine and became successful physicians. After studying at Leyden he became physician to the court of the Prince of Orange and, at the nomination of the Prince, he was awarded the Oxford M.D. Elected a fellow of the College of Physicians in 1677 he became a Harveian orator. The Annals of the College describe him as 'a person of great skill in the practice of medicine'.

Communis Europae Praeceptor (the teacher of all Europe) — such was the tribute of his Swiss pupil Albrecht von Haller, to Herman Boerhaave of Leyden. That von Haller's description was no exaggeration can plainly be seen from the subsequent advances made in the countries to which Boerhaave's more brilliant pupils returned from Leyden. These included Carl Linnaeus to Uppsala, Albrecht von Haller to Göttingen, Alexander Monro (and others) to Edinburgh, and Gerhard van Swieten to Vienna. In the case of Edinburgh the return of the Scottish postgraduate students from Leyden virtually transformed the medical school. In the same way van Swieten founded the old Vienna Medical School and von Haller the medical faculty at Göttingen.

In his impressive volume, *Herman Boerhaave, the Man and His Work,* Prof. G. A. Lindeboom of Amsterdam provides a striking introduction to the character and immense industry of this astonishing genius. The son of a Reformed minister in a parish near Leyden, he entered Leyden University as a theological student. His father's early death and several other factors, however, caused him to change to Medicine. One of these considerations was his hope to combine (much as a medical missionary does) the work of minister and doctor.

In 1701 Boerhaave became Reader in Medicine at Leyden at the age of 32 and then in 1709 both Professor of Medicine and Professor of Botany. In addition (incredible as it may seem — though all subjects were less specialized in those days) he was appointed Professor of Chemistry in 1718! The records indicate that he industriously set to work to make his teaching effective in all three of his departments! It was his role as botanist, which first attracted Linnaeus, and he much improved and extended the famous Physic Garden of the university.

Boerhaave had earlier been greatly impressed by the writings of Thomas Sydenham, and especially with the latter's empirical attitude to disease and the individual patient. On being appointed to St. Caecilian's Hospital in Leyden he became a pioneer teacher of clinical medicine. At first he had only 12 beds at St. Caecilian's but he re-introduced bedside teaching and laid down clinical attitudes to patient care to be followed by his disciples throughout Europe. The chief medical writings of this prodigious worker, besides transcripts of his lectures, were the two Latin textbooks — *The Institutes of Medicine* and *The Aphorisms concerning the Knowledge and Care of Diseases*. These were printed in many Latin editions, translated into a number of languages and had a world-wide circulation.

G. A. Lindeboom, discussing the strengths of this great teacher writes: 'Boerhaave had experienced a secret intercourse with God. However heavy were his tasks for the day, each morning he spent an hour in prayer and meditation. In that hour he drew from the source of divine grace the strength for his Christian attitude during the bustle and annoyance of the day. . . . His harmonious and equable personality was undoubtedly not only due to his heredity and environment, but was also the fruit of an inner, spiritual life, which mostly remained hidden from his pupils, patients and friends.'

BOERHAAVE'S DISCIPLES

Of the many eminent men who were influenced by Boerhaave in the countries of Europe, two may be mentioned here — Carl Linnaeus and Albrecht von Haller. Both shared many personal resemblances to him in character and outlook.

Carl von Linné (Linnaeus) was the son of a Swedish Lutheran pastor, who desired that his son also should follow him into the service of the Church. However, Carl turned to the natural sciences and Medicine in the belief that God had chosen him to explore natural phenomena. In the process he became the father of natural history. He realized the importance of the reproductive systems in plants and built his classification of the vegetable world on them. At this period the botanical department of a university was part of the medical faculty, and interest was centred in collecting the raw herbs needed by the apothecaries for their medicinal products. For this reason Linnaeus had qualified medically so that he could subsequently go on to his botanical studies. On his return to Sweden, Linnaeus sought to reform the medical education of the University of Uppsala. He also attempted to classify diseases — in his *Genera Morborum* — into a pattern of genera and species though, when this was applied by William Cullen in Edinburgh it was soon found to be inappropriate to the natural history of disease.

Linnaeus' simple faith in God is illustrated by the description of his reaction when visiting England in springtime and seeing a gorse bush in full bloom. He then and there knelt down and offered thanksgiving to God for such a wonderful sight.

Another prominent disciple of Boerhaave, Albrecht von Haller, was from Berne, Switzerland and was a devout Christian. He soon became one of those men of genius who have simultaneously shone in several different fields of human endeavour — in this case as botanist, physiologist, poet and novelist. After studying at Tübingen and Leyden and pursuing postgraduate work in London and Paris he was appointed to the newly founded University of Göttingen. There he concurrently held the chairs of anatomy, botany and medicine. He remained for 17 years teaching and quietly helping to mould the medical faculty of Göttingen into being the 'Leyden' of Germany. It was here also that he did his best experimental work and wrote some 13,000 scientific papers! He also established botanical gardens and a number of churches. He wrote the first textbook devoted to physiology alone and also a flora of his native Switzerland. His physiological treatise became expanded into a massive eight-volume work published in 1757, so that von Haller may be regarded as the founder of modern physiology. Among other findings he confirmed Glisson's speculation that irritability was an inherent property of muscle tissue. His most famous poem was *Die Alpen* (1729) which reflects the glory of God in the majesty of the Swiss mountain scenery. Although he was an evangelical Protestant and inclined towards Pietism, at times he wrote more like a disciple of the rationalist Enlightenment. It has been suggested of him that at the same time 'he thought as a rationalist and believed as a sincere Christian'.

Besides Albrecht von Haller, others of Boerhaave's students came to exercise immense influence in the countries which they subsequently served. For example, two able Dutchmen, who (because of their devout Catholicism) could not have risen in professional rank in the Reformation University of Leyden, reached European fame from their beneficent work in Vienna. Gerhard van Swieten was first appointed physician-in-ordinary to the Empress Marie Theresa of Austria. He was soon invited to lecture on Medicine in the University. He did this to such good purpose that he rapidly came to have immense authority in the Austrian medical profession. He gradually introduced to the medical faculty the new scientific clinical approach and bedside teaching of Boerhaave, and in the end completely transformed the antiquated Viennese School.

Becoming a favourite of the Empress, van Swieten gained increasing administrative importance. Eventually — not without opposition from the senior members of the faculty and city's doctors — he boldly introduced reforms which transported all the features characteristic of Leyden. For example, he set up a well-stocked herb garden and a chemical laboratory on the Boerhaave pattern. But more importantly he introduced the effective teaching of clinical medicine by having twelve beds, six for men and six for women, set aside in the City Hospital for teaching the students. He then reorganized — by imperial decree — the teaching institutions and total structure of the medical profession. Also, having been made the director, he transformed the public library in Vienna into the most up-to-date and scientific in Europe at that time.

Among the most valuable legacies of van Swieten to Viennese Medicine were, first, the gradual completion of his *Commentary on the Aphorisms of Boerhaave* which he had started as a student in Leyden and which was published after his death. Then, most productive of all, was his bringing a younger clinician from Leyden, Anton de Haen, to lead the most important medical clinic in Vienna.

The character and abilities of Anton de Haen were ideally suited to the position which he came to occupy. He was a born clinician and a born teacher. He not only continued but advanced the teachings in clinical medicine begun by Boerhaave and van Swieten. Vienna came to attract an increasing number of medical students and postgraduates from all over Europe. He began a fashion for preserving full case histories, reports of successful treatments and reports of the results of the Clinics. These were published in 1758 in eighteen volumes under the title *Ratio Medendi in Nosocomio Practico (Therapeutics in Hospital Practice)*. De Haen was restricted to no one system of Medicine and the importance of his publications consisted in their open-minded scientific empiricism. The outcome of van Swieten's and de Haen's work was that the Viennese School of Medicine in outlook and approach became the pattern of the new Western Medicine.

SOME ENGLISH PHYSICIANS AND SURGEONS

An English physician who claims attention is William Heberden. When Dr. Samuel Johnson was afflicted by his last illness, he was asked what physician he had called. He replied, 'Dr. Heberden, ultimus Romanorum, the last of our learned physicians'. Heberden had built up a very successful practice in London. He took careful notes of his own clinical observations and from them he wrote a series of *Commentaries on the History and Cure of Diseases*. These were written largely for his son, William Heberden the younger. Heberden learned from his own experience and did not depend greatly on the writings of others. His accounts of angina pectoris, chicken pox, 'Heberden's nodes' of the fingers, and night blindness are classic descriptions of these conditions. That of angina pectoris which was first published in the *Medical Transactions of the Royal College of Physicians* (1772) is so accurate and graphic that it might with very few alterations be published in a modern volume. By the time he wrote his *Commentaries* he had observed no less than 100 cases.

While others had come very near to realizing that chickenpox was a distinct entity from smallpox, it was Heberden who finally made the clear-cut distinction in a paper he read in 1767, the gist of which was also published in the *Commentaries*. He recognized that an attack of chickenpox did not confer immunity to smallpox infection, although he realized that it gave life-long immunity to a further attack of the same disease. He raised his voice against the absurdly complicated prescriptions which had dogged Medicine from medieval times. Some of these had contained up to 54 ingredients! Earlier criticisms had been brought against these absurd and useless concoctions by Culpeper in the mid-17th century. Heberden delivered the *coup de grâce* in a monograph *Essay on Mithridatium and Antitheriaca (Essay on Antidotes to Poisons)*.

A prominent surgeon at the time was Charles Bell, who is still recalled today because his name is associated with Bell's palsy and the long thoracic nerve of Bell. He had a brother John who was a surgeon in Edinburgh. They were the sons of an Episcopalian clergyman who died when Charles was only five years old. After qualifying at Edinburgh Charles left for London and founded a school of anatomy. He also lectured to artists on human anatomy and from these lectures emerged his volume on *The Anatomy of Expression* (1806). He himself was an able illustrator and he illustrated most of his works with his own sketches. Working with Wilson as partner he took over the famous Windmill Street School of Anatomy. In 1811 he published *A New Idea of the Anatomy of the Brain and Nervous System* in which he noted that stimulation of the anterior root of the spinal nerves produced muscular contraction but stimulation of the posterior roots did not. This work was brought to the attention of Magendie who then formulated the idea of motor and sensory nerves. Bell had similarly described the facial and trigeminal nerves of the face but it remained for his own student Mayo to recognize clearly that the former was motor and the latter sensory. In both cases Bell vehemently maintained the priority of his own understanding of the situation. In 1814 Bell was appointed surgeon to the Middlesex Hospital and in 1815, after news had come through of the battle of Waterloo, he and his brother-in-law John Shaw rushed over to the battlefield. Although they arrived at the scene of carnage several days after the battle was over, they both set to work to operate on the wounded of both sides. In spite of all that there was to do, he took time to sketch some of the appalling wounds he encountered. In 1830 there appeared a further volume of the *Nervous System of the Human Body* which has been described as a medical classic. The newer ideas of nerve function were by now generally accepted. In 1836 he returned to Edinburgh to take up the chair of surgery there. His private letters reveal Bell as a deeply religious man. He was approached by the Archbishop of Canterbury and the Bishop of London to contribute a thesis to the trust fund set up under the will of the Earl of Bridgwater to illustrate some aspect of 'the power, wisdom and goodness of God as manifested in the Creation'. Bell chose the human hand as the subject of his thesis and produced a volume the full title of which is *The Hand; its Mechanisms and Vital Endowments, as evincing design, and illustrating the power, wisdom and goodness of God* (1833).

A physician, Caleb Parry, was the original describer of hyperthyroidism. He was a pupil of John Hunter and settled as a physician in Bath. His account of eight cases of hyperthyroidism was published posthumously in 1825, ten years before Graves published his account of three cases. Parry was also the first to describe facial hemiatrophy (1814) and congenital idiopathic dilatation of the colon (1825). He kept careful records of his patients and in 1788 read a paper before a small country medical society in which he attributed angina pectoris to disease of the coronary arteries. He had wide general interests, acquired a farm and wrote on sheep breeding. Among his last writings was an essay on the character of Hamlet. Parry was a sincere Christian, the son of a scholarly dissenting minister, and was educated at the Warrington academy and at Edinburgh.

Theophile Hyacinth Laennec invented the stethoscope, which has become as much the symbol of the doctor as the sickle was of the agricultural worker. Laennec's original instrument, however, looked more like an old fashioned fetal stethoscope. He described the sounds he heard with it and correlated these with the underlying pulmonary pathology. His work was thus the foundation for the modern advances in the care of chest diseases. Laennec was both a sincere Catholic and a Royalist. He was a man of gentle utterance but spoke very much to the point.

THE QUAKER CONTRIBUTION

The doctor members of the Religious Society of Friends (Quakers) were true members of the age of the Enlightenment. Their enquiring minds and scientific interests ranged over the entire field of human knowledge. Their religious concern for all people led them beyond conventional medical practice to instigate practical measures to combat the social wrongs that undermined the health of the people. At the same time they were active members of their Society, often serving as clerks, elders and ministers. Two of the most influential among them were John Fothergill and John Coakley Lettsom.

Fothergill was perhaps the more eminent. He gave a clear description of diphtheria, although he did not differentiate the condition from what we should call a streptococcal sore throat, nor did he give the disease its present name. Fothergill described what he had seen during an epidemic in London under the title *An Account of the Sore Throat attended with Ulcers* (1748). He carefully portrayed the general condition and the appearance of the fauces. He realized that the slough covered an ulcer and described the fetid material which was discharged from the nostril. In 1773 he also described 'tic douloureux', of which he had come across 16 cases, though, again, he did not give it this actual name.

He was not only an outstanding consultant physician but also busied himself in prison reform and the improvement of medical education. Throughout his life he remained an active and consistent Quaker and three times acted as clerk to the yearly meetings of Quakers in London. He had many contacts with America and used his efforts to try to prevent the war which eventually broke out between the colonies and the motherland.

Fothergill was also concerned about the problem of communicating modern advances among the physicians. In 1752 he was a leading member of a group of London physicians who agreed to 'meet together from time to time in order to discuss the prevalent diseases and their means of cure and for their mutual improvement in the practice of their profession'. This followed the example of a similar society in the Edinburgh of their student days and developed into the Medical Society of London. The group published a series of bound volumes containing their discussions and the papers read to the Society. It was at Fothergill's expense that the first of this series of six volumes was published under the title of *Medical Observations and Inquiries*.

John Coakley Lettsom inherited something of the outlook of Fothergill, whose pupil he had been. He too was a competent caring physician deeply conscious of the social needs of his day and showing a spirit of kindliness and cooperation in treating the sick. He was one of the earliest of the physicians, as distinct from the apothecaries, to visit the patients in their homes. He was interested in botany and founded a botanic garden at his home in the then salubrious area of Camberwell Green. He described alcoholism as a medical condition and helped to launch the Royal Humane Society for reviving the apparently dead from drowning. He was the prime mover in founding the sea bathing infirmary at Margate which was especially designed for children suffering from scrofula (tuberculous cervical glands). In this way he became the father of the many sanatoria of the next century. He was also instrumental, with Fothergill, in founding the distinguished and still active Medical Society of London. Among papers which he himself presented at the Society's meetings were 'The cause of pain in rheumatism' and 'The defence of inoculation.' However, after Jenner's work became known he supported vaccination, since he believed that inoculation, although it protected the individual, probably contributed to the spread of smallpox in the community.

This influential Quaker circle extended across the Atlantic to America. Indeed, many in the Society of Friends had left the homeland for a country where they could worship according to their beliefs in greater freedom. The medical pioneer Benjamin Rush was deeply influenced by Quaker thought and took an active part in founding the first medical school in America at Philadelphia, himself occupying the chair of the Institute of Medicine. He was regarded as the outstanding American physician of his time. He described yellow fever and also drew attention to focal sepsis. His description of dengue, yellow fever (which he called the 'bilious remitting fever' in his publication) and his treatise on insanity are classics. He was a pioneer of the temperance movement, advocated prison reforms and the abolition of public and capital punishment. He also championed education for girls and proposed a theory of education which gave greater freedom to children. Later he became increasingly broad in his ecclesiastical sympathies, but remained deeply religious. His signature appears on the American Declaration of Independence.

In the 19th century the Quakers continued to make a substantial contribution to Medicine. One cause of the channelling of their abilities into the medical profession and social services was undoubtedly the fact that legal restrictions (not to be relaxed until late in the century) closed so many other doors. Also, their seriousness and sense of honesty inspired them to search for the truth, and their sturdy sense of independence made them question authority in all departments of life. Added to this was their strong attitude of compassion. Space prevents more than a few additional references to other members of this remarkable community.

Thomas Hodgkin was born into a Quaker family. When in France he visited Laennec the inventor of the stethoscope, and brought one back with him. He was appointed demonstrator in morbid anatomy and curator of the museum at Guy's Hospital, but was never appointed one of its physicians. The reason may have been that when one of his friends was going to North America he had asked him to enquire how the natives were treated by the Hudson Bay Company. The report was unfavourable and Hodgkin communicated it to Harrison, who was on the board both of the Hudson Bay Company and of Guy's Hospital. This probably prejudiced Hodgkin's chances of obtaining the appointment of physician to the Hospital, although he continued his lectures in pathology and various other interests. He set a high standard in pathology by his catalogue of the Guy's reports and post-mortem records. He was a founder member of the Senate of the University of London. For many years he was secretary of the Royal Geographical Association and was interested in the emancipation of the slaves and their resettlement after they had been freed.

In 1828 appeared his 'Essay on Medical Education', and in 1832 his

'Hints Relative to Cholera in London'. His most famous paper, describing lymphadenoma also appeared in 1832 in the *Transactions of the Royal Medical and Chirurgical Society* and was entitled 'A Series of Cases of Contemporaneous Enlargement of the Spleen and Absorbing Glands', which today we should call lymph nodes. Some 30 years later in 1865 Dr. Samuel Wilks, also of Guy's Hospital, independently discovered this same condition and named it Hodgkin's disease. The microscope had come into general use by Wilks' time and on re-examining micro-scopically Hodgkin's original specimens he found that not all of them had in fact been Hodgkin's disease. Hodgkin also produced *Lectures on the Morbid Anatomy of Serous and Mucous Membranes* (1836).

Another devout Quaker, Jonathan Hutchinson, a surgeon to the London Hospital from 1859-1883, was a man of many interests – general surgery, ophthalmology, dermatology and neurology. It was he who first described 'Hutchinson's teeth', a sign of congenital syphilis, in a paper in the *British Medical Journal* of 1861. Little Sarah W. was a patient in the London Hospital. She was 11 years old and had an intractable ulcer of her leg. Could it be 'an inherited taint of syphilis'? Following up this idea, he looked at her teeth and found that her upper incisors were of a characteristic shape. It was also Hutchinson who first described the dilated pupil found in certain serious head injuries and which is important in showing on which side haemorrhage has taken place. In 1866 Jacobsen suggested that it should be called 'Hutchinson's pupil'.

THE EMERGENCE OF SPECIALTIES

In the 18th century came the emergence of the specialist doctor. Surgeons were becoming more established as specialists in their own right, rather than as 'technicians' doing the bidding of the physicians. In 1745 they broke away from the Barbers' Company and formed their own 'incorpora-tion'. 'Man midwives' were also becoming more recognized. One factor in their acceptance was the publication of details of the obstetric forceps which had hitherto been kept a family secret by the French Huguenot family, the Chamberlens.

The apothecaries were fast becoming the forerunners of the general practitioners and, as such, had to fight for their standing with the members and fellows of the Royal College of Physicians. John Mason Good formed an association of apothecaries to protect those practising from both the physicians and the commercial interests of the drug manufacturers. Good, the son of a Congregational Minister, who had studied Medicine, wrote on a variety of topics including a four-volume work entitled *'A study of Medicine'* (1803). His religious interests are shown by his writing commentaries on *The Song of Songs* and *The Psalms,* containing his own translations.

The term 'orthopedia' was coined by Nicolas André from the Greek words *orthos,* straight and *pedes,* child. Increasing interest was shown in both orthopaedics and paediatrics and notable in the latter field was Rosen von Rosenstein. His book on the subject was the most progressive which had yet been written. Rosenstein, whose mother came from a deeply religious family, commenced his studies as a theological student preparing for the ministry in the Lutheran church. He later changed to Medicine and after qualification was appointed to the chair of Natural History at Uppsala where Carl von Linné (Linnaeus) (see p. 74) occupied the chair of medicine. Much to the benefit of both medicine and botany they were later able to exchange their professorial chairs.

A London physician, Michael Underwood, wrote a slim volume entitled *Treatise on the Diseases of Children,* which went through 17 editions. Like so many other medical books it increased in size with each edition and ended up as a three-volume work. Underwood had studied under a well known surgeon of St. George's Hospital, Caesar Hawkins. On qualifying as a surgeon he was appointed to the British Lying-in Hospital, and after a time he devoted himself to midwifery and, especially, diseases of childhood. 'Underwood with more perseverance than most people, had kept a daily record of his life, interspersed with meditations on various subjects, mostly religious, for over sixty years. It extended to over 122 volumes(!)'

Dermatology also began to attract more attention. Mention has been made of Robert Willan in discussing the dispensary movement. 'He was the first physician of this country to arrange diseases of the skin in a clear and intelligible manner and to fix their nomenclature on a satisfactory and classical basis.' In 1790 he was awarded the Fothergill gold medal for his classification of skin diseases. Being a classical scholar he had drawn upon his knowledge of the Greek, Latin and Arabic names for eruptive disorders of the skin. Between 1798 and 1808 he published his magnum opus *Description and Treatment of Cutaneous Diseases,* the last part of this work appearing after his death. His other medical interests included the effects of climate on disease in London. He was greatly concerned about and active in promoting the health and welfare of the poor. In 1782 he published a *History of the Ministry of Jesus Christ,* compiled from the accounts of the four Evangelists in the New Testament.

In addition to preventive medicine, anaesthesia and surgery – which will be given special attention in the following chapter – there were two further areas of study in which Christians were prominent among the pioneers. These were physiology and psychiatry.

PHYSIOLOGY

Stephen Hales, an Anglican minister in Teddington, although not medically qualified, conducted a series of significant physiological investigations, for example by 'inserting a brass cannula connected to a glass tube into an artery of a horse to measure the height to which the blood rose'. He released measured volumes of blood at regular intervals and measured the falling levels of blood pressure thus produced. His experiments are in the same class as those of Harvey. He described his experiments in the quaintly worded *'Statical Essays containing Hemostaticks'* (1733). His results demonstrated the close interrelationship between blood flow, blood velocity, blood pressure and cardiac output. He had previously studied plant physiology and published his results as *Vegetable Statics*. Later he was awarded the Copley gold medal of the Royal Society for his researches into urinary calculi. He was the inventor of artificial ventilation and when his windmill ventilator was installed in Newgate prison it is said to have reduced the mortality by 75%. In spite of all his scientific experiments he did not neglect his primary vocation and also showed practical common sense in many directions. For example, he enlarged the churchyard, put a lantern on the church tower, supervised the building of a new aisle to the church towards which he himself contributed £200, and helped to secure a better water supply for his parishioners. Like so many of the natural scientists of that period he regarded his work as demonstrating the handiwork of the Divine Architect, whose wisdom was to be seen in 'so just a symmetry of parts, such innumerable beauties and harmony'.

A versatile Italian priest, Abbé Spallanzani, also conducted a variety of experiments in the fields of botany, physiology and geology. He obtained samples of the gastric juice by attaching sponges to cords which were then swallowed. When they were retrieved he demonstrated that digestion was not a process of putrefaction as had been thought. He appropriately used the microscope in his researches. A century before Pasteur he had really already undermined the theory of spontaneous generation by showing that organic materials when heated in sealed containers did not undergo fermentation. He also showed that seminal fluid was essential to germination of the ovum and he suggested the possibilities of artificial insemination.

Advances in physiology, however, did not come rapidly until the second half of the 19th century, but one outstanding worker was to do his important work early in the first half. Marshall Hall was the fourth son of Robert Hall, a cotton manufacturer in Nottingham who was the first commercially to use chlorine in bleaching. His father was a strong Methodist and generous philanthropist, and the son shared to the full in both traits. Marshall Hall was medically trained in Edinburgh and, on qualifying, spent several months in the chief medical centres of the Continent. He then developed a large practice first in Nottingham and later in central London.

Hall used every available moment and especially the late night hours for his physiological research. A list of his discoveries — considering his busy practice — is impressive. He opposed the contemporary practice of blood-letting, and demonstrated the anatomy and physiology of the capillary blood vessels. His chief discovery was reflex nerve action, which he demonstrated in the newt. He also introduced a number of other advances and their practical applications, for example the Marshall Hall method of artificial respiration, which saved many lives. In private life Hall was the energetic supporter of many important reforming movements, for example those to end flogging in the Army and the remnants of slavery in the Americas.

A distinguished physiologist of the late years of the 19th century was Michael Foster. Born of nonconformist yeoman ancestors he graduated in classics and then proceeded to qualify in Medicine at University College Hospital, London. After a short period of study in Paris he set up in practice in Huntingdon, but in 1867 his former teacher William Sharpey invited him to join the Physiology Department at University College. Two years later he was appointed Professor of Physiology there and subsequently Professor of Physiology in Cambridge. An able organizer and administrator, he inspired many pupils in various fields of physiology. He was a leading member in the formation of the Physiological Society in 1875. He also founded the *Journal of Physiology* in 1878 and wrote one of the standard textbooks for students which has been described as the 'first authoritative textbook in the English language on physiology'. In 1900 he became Liberal Member of Parliament for the University of London. Shortly afterwards he gave a series of lectures in America which were subsequently published as *Lectures on the History of Physiology,* but he then retired from professional work. He had been interested in the physiology of the heart, and seeing that small pieces of detached heart muscle continued to beat, he deduced that the heart beat must be a specific property of heart muscle. He also suggested that the transmission of impulses from nerve to muscle must involve electrical forces.

Michael Foster was a Baptist and this had prevented him from entering the University of Cambridge as an undergraduate; he had therefore turned to University College, London, which had been formed to break down religious barriers to entry on a professional career. Ackerknecht quotes the Baptist Foster as an example of how German Jews, English Dissenters and French Protestants became 19th century pioneers of modern medicine and science (p. 2).

PSYCHIATRY

For long psychiatry did not emerge as a fully fledged specialty in its own right and many of those who were suffering from mental illness were still being treated by the clergy rather than by doctors. Also the prevailing custom was to make use of a private 'madhouse' for inpatient treatment. Although many of these institutions were well run according to the standards of the time, others left much to be desired. The financial gain of the proprietor could so easily overrule the interests of the patient, especially as at that time the definition of what constituted 'madness' was much less precise than it is today. Also there was general acceptance of certain forms of treatment which can only be called brutal. For example, even George III, his mind deranged by porphyria, was put into a straight-jacket, knocked down, and otherwise severely maltreated. Earlier in the century that doughty outspoken dissenter Daniel Defoe had lifted his pen against the abuses of the private madhouse in his *True Born Englishman*. In the London area the poor 'insane' were usually admitted to the Bethlem Hospital, to which the well-to-do flocked as visitors to be amused by the patients' antics. As Bethlem (shortened from Bethlehem and popularized as 'Bedlam') was in any case insufficient to meet all the demand, in 1751 a small committee set about forming St. Luke's Hospital for the 'insane' which was opened in Moorfields, London.

Among the Christian clergymen-physicians who made the beginnings of advance in the understanding of mental illness were the following. Richard Blackmore, a member of the Society for the Propagation of the Gospel in America and physician to the court, accurately described the manic-depressive's swings of mood. He also distinguished what today we should call neurotic from psychotic depression. Lewis Southcombe, 'a country clergyman who had studied physic in London and combined the cure of souls with that of bodies', expressed himself against the cruder forms of treatment of his day. He did his best to dispel the aura of disgrace and shame that centred around mental illness. 'Why should not one form of distemper invade us as well as any other?' Hugh Farmer, a minister of religion at Walthamstow, boldly attacked witch hunting. He suggested that the demoniacs in the New Testament were either 'mad, melancholy or epileptic persons'. His essay was 'a major blow to superstition and in this sense was an opportune apology for psychiatry'. Francis Willis was a clergyman, who had started to practise Medicine even before he gained a qualification in 1759. He became a physician at Lincoln Hospital, which he had helped to found, and later became respected for his skill in handling mental cases. His fame was such that he was invited to attend George III in spite of the opposition of the royal physicians of the time. He worked on the principle that 'if theory was lacking or unrewarding, then plain common sense must be used' and he was the first to apply these principles in the treatment of psychiatric patients.

Charles Moore, rector of Cuxton in Kent, published in 1790 *A Full Inquiry into the Subject of Suicide*. He concluded that the question of whether all victims of suicide were necessarily insane must remain in dispute. His detached and humane attitude was unusual in a day when religious people tended to regard suicide as a sin. William Falconer, a physician at Bath, was a member of Fothergill's circle, and wrote on theological subjects. He foreshadowed the psychosomatic concept in his *Dissertation on the Influence of the Passions upon Disorders of the Body,* for which he was awarded the Fothergill silver medal. He also advocated spa treatment. This versatile worker was one in whom 'the noble ideals of Fothergill had found a true response'. Another worker in this field was William Pargeteer who was both a doctor and clergyman. He wrote on *Observations of Maniacal Disorders,* a volume that has been highly praised. He realized that 'the chief reliance in the cure of Insanity must rather be on management than medicine'.

A major step by one of the Christians who were concerned to care for the mentally ill was taken by a Quaker tea merchant, William Tuke, who founded The Retreat, York. Hannah Mills, a member of the Society of Friends at York, had been admitted to the York Asylum and died there. The Quakers had been refused permission to visit her and suspected that she had been illtreated. It was this that made Tuke lay a proposal before the quarterly meeting of the Society that they should found 'a retired habitation . . . for the members of our society and others in profession with us, who may be in a state of lunacy, or so deranged in mind as to require such provision'. They raised a subscription and launched The Retreat in 1796. The name was chosen 'to convey the idea of what such an institution should be, namely a place in which the unhappy might obtain a refuge, a quiet haven in which the shattered bark might find the means of reparation or safety'. Little stress was laid on drugs or medicines but encouragement was given to warm baths, a liberal diet, suitable amusements and reading. Corporal punishment and chains were banned. Thomas Fowler, a nonconformist though not a Quaker, was appointed as first physician to the Retreat.

Although the work of William Tuke of York, and about the same time Philippe Pinel in Paris, had graphically called attention to the appalling conditions in which psychiatric cases were at that time being kept, the appropriate further changes were still slow to come. There was even a good deal of public opinion which was opposed to the abolition of the prisonlike conditions and mechanical restraints of the asylums.

Edward Long Fox was a Quaker physician with advanced views on the treatment of mental illness. In 1794 he took charge of a small Quaker mental asylum near Bristol. He himself had been influenced by the Frenchman Pinel who was the son of a country practitioner and who had begun his career as a student of divinity. In 1804 Fox built an entirely new hospital at Brislington where every patient had a separate room opening on to a court in which were kept tame silver pheasants and doves. Fox encouraged his patients to look after these birds and also gave them other suitable employment in the house and grounds whenever their condition permitted. He would allow no one to stay in bed except when physically ill. Common rooms and entertainments of various kinds were provided, but he insisted on rigid segregation of the sexes. Even in the chapel, which was served by visiting clergy of all denominations, women sat on one side and men on the other.

While there were other individual physicians who here and there made small advances, the significant advances in the specialty of psychiatry had to await the second half of the 19th century. During these earlier times a considerable proportion of the active support for the pioneers who built and administered better asylums came from the Christian Churches which were socially concerned. The Pietists of Germany and Scandinavia, following the pattern set by the philanthropic Hermann Francke of Halle, were specially active in meeting all forms of need by funding the appropriate institutions, including mental hospitals.

Towards the close of the 19th century the Protestant Churches of the Netherlands became specially active in these respects. Lucas Lindeboom, a professor of theology in the college of the Gereformerde Kerken (the Free Reformed Churches) at Kampen, claimed that so far the churches as a whole had failed in their duty to the mentally ill, the mentally deficient and all forms of handicapped persons. As there was but a small response to his appeal, in 1884 he founded the Vereeniging tot Christelijk Verzorging van Krankzinnigen (the Society for Christian Support for the Sick in Mind) which in turn inspired the formation of similar societies for other forms of handicap. The original society was responsible for the establishment of five great mental hospitals between the years 1886 and 1910. The State Church (Hervormde Kerk) was subsequently led to found similar institutions under its own auspices.

In Denmark fruitful pioneer work was done by Adolph Sell who founded the 'colony' of Filadelfia, a residential community for epileptics. Success with this group of patients led to an extension of admissions to the colony of those suffering other severe nervous diseases. Sell was succeeded as superintendent of the colony by Hans Jacob Schon who added a psychiatric department under the name Dianalund Nervesanatorium. Schon who was Chairman of the Christian Medical Association of Denmark (1929-1947) brought inspiration along these lines to doctors in the whole of Scandinavia. For example, in Norway it became possible for whole families to be resident in one of the houses within the colony during the period of long stay treatment for one of the parents.

THE CLERGYMAN-PHYSICIAN

In this setting it is relevant to refer to the services rendered by the clergy to Medicine in some other countries. In areas where communications were poor and there was a dearth of qualified doctors, there was a distinct place for the educated, partially trained, layman who could give simple medical treatment. The German physician Johann Peter Frank, who successively practised in Germany, Austria and Russia and held appointments in two Courts and five universities, expounded a similar idea in his *A System of Complete Medical Polity*. This treatise advocated something approaching a complete national health service with priest-doctors and medical assistants in the remote rural areas where the population was very small. It was published in six principal volumes and three supplementary volumes.

Robert Heller in an article in *Medical History* has discussed 'Priest-Doctors as a Rural Health Service in the Age of the Enlightenment'. Much thought and discussion, mainly in Protestant countries, was given to this source of auxiliary medical aid in sparsely populated areas. Heller discusses Johann Peter Frank's address on the value of priest-doctors before the University of Vienna, given just before his departure to Russia where he attempted to organize better medical services. Only in Sweden — where Linnaeus had already advocated a similar idea — were arrangements implemented for elementary medical training for the Lutheran clergy of the remote country districts. On the whole, however, the project was not a success, except in the case of a few of the clergy who had natural gifts for the task. Although critical of some of his own Church's practices (he regarded himself as a loyal catholic) Frank advocated that the clergy should be trained in Medicine so that they could practise the dual rôle of doctor and priest in rural areas.

James Clegg, a Presbyterian minister working in Chapel-en-le-Frith in the Peak District, was an example of a man who was active both medically and theologically. He had to take up farming to supplement his meagre clerical income and also started to treat the poor of his area. But increasingly the more affluent of the parish sought his advice. It must be remembered how ineffective most of the treatments of those days were and how few were the investigations that even the orthodox doctors could bring to bear on their cases. When antagonists threatened to prosecute him, claiming that he was using his privileged position to obtain patients, he applied *in absentia* to Aberdeen University for a degree to practise. His successful application was supported by Dr. Nettleton of Halifax, Dr. Dixon of Bolton and Dr. Latham of Findern, of whom the latter two were also combining the functions of dissenting minister and doctor. Clegg's diaries have recently been edited and published; they record the cases he dealt with and the prevailing local social conditions. The concept of medical auxiliary assistants was to find a more welcome application in the 20th century Third World (see chapter 13).

As the scope of Medicine widened, and as the particular needs of patients had to be more efficiently met, so the profession improvised and specialized. Most of the specialities were developed in the late 19th and 20th centuries. They have continued to proliferate and have become more specialized within themselves. It is beyond the scope of this study to pursue their developments in detail.

CHAPTER 7

UNDERSTANDING INFECTION, RELIEVING PAIN AND SAFER SURGERY

THE latter part of the 19th century has become known as 'the age of miracles', especially in the department of surgery. The chief barriers to what could be done had been (i) the daunting mortality in the general hospitals resulting from sepsis, (ii) the acute pain of major operations and (iii) the prevention, or replacement, of severe blood-loss. In the 19th century, at last, sepsis and pain were overcome. The full conquest of the third barrier had to await the horrors of World Wars I and II. The highlights in the story have been graphically described in many forms and places. The essentials will, however, bear brief repetition.

Looking back from the vantage point of today's skilled surgical techniques it remains a matter for wonder that the breakthrough came so long after the first hopeful beginnings. For at various periods of history gifted pioneers have from time to time pointed the way. As already described in Chapter 3, William of Saliceto in the 13th century had dressed his patients' wounds with white of egg and rosewater and achieved good results. He had been followed by his disciples Theodore Borgognoni and Henri de Mondeville who both taught and emphasized cleanliness. They used wine or dry dressings and believed that, ideally, wounds should all heal by first intention. Their example was forgotten until in the 16th century Ambroîse Paré dramatically rediscovered the conservative treatment of wounds on the French battlefields. Again, the way forward was not taken and could not fully be followed until the nature of infection by microorganisms came to be understood and the tyranny of blind belief in 'spontaneous generation' had been broken.

INFECTION

As early as 1546, in a book entitled *De Contagione,* Girolamo Fracastoro had suggested that among the causes of illness were 'seeds of disease which multiply rapidly and propagate their life'. His contemporaries, however, remained unconvinced, especially because these 'seeds' could not be seen nor their direct effects plainly demonstrated. Later, a Dutch linen merchant, Anthony van Leeuwenhoek, began to grind his own lenses and spend his free time with his microscopes. Although the magnification was not very great he was able to see and describe red blood cells, spermatozoa and microorganisms from his own mouth — 'little animals, more numerous than all the people in the Netherlands'. Again, not much purposive notice of his work was taken at that time.

A beginning, however, was made in 1773 by Charles White, a Manchester surgeon practising also as an obstetrician, who published a book on the management of obstetric cases. He greatly reduced the incidence of puerperal fever in his wards by requiring cleanliness and proper ventilation in the labour wards and recommending the use of disinfectants post partum. It seems, however, that he had not fully grasped the nature of puerperal infection for he did not insist on strict cleanliness of the hands of everyone who was to be in contact with the patient.

But in 1795 several practical steps were taken by an Aberdeen obstetrician, Alexander Gordon, who came nearer to the solution. Worried by the very high rates of mortality from puerperal fever following so many of the maternity cases in the wards, he instituted a regime of strict cleanliness on the part of all coming into contact with patients. The result was a significant lowering in the incidence of the fever. He went on to advocate that all nurses and physicians attending patients affected with puerperal fever ought to wash themselves and get their apparel properly fumigated.

Some years later, in 1847, the Hungarian Ignaz Philipp Semmelweis noticed in an obstetric hospital in Vienna that the incidence of puerperal fever in the wards attended by students was considerably greater than in the midwives' ward. He therefore ordered every student to bathe his hands in a solution of chlorinated lime before examining a patient. The incidence of sepsis immediately fell from 18% to under 2%. Unfortunately, because of the jealousy of some of his senior colleagues, his measures were not properly taken up. He was put in charge of a hospital in Pest, which had recently suffered an outbreak of puerperal fever, and proceeded to reduce the annual mortality rate there to under 1%. But, in spite of this, stubborn opposition continued and he died a broken-hearted man. It was not until Pasteur's convincing proofs of the error of 'spontaneous generation' and the fact that blood, meat and other fluids do not putrefy if they are preserved from external contamination, that the great liberation finally came.

Louis Pasteur was professor of chemistry successively at Strasbourg, Lille and Paris. His publications concerning microorganisms put an end to the humoral theory of disease, the practice of blood letting, and the prevailing belief in spontaneous generation, and set in train a veritable hunt for microorganisms in all manner of diseases. His active mind investigated one problem after another, including diseases of wine, of insects and of man. Influenced by the work of Jenner, he introduced a graded attenuated vaccine for the treatment of rabies. In 1888 the Institut Pasteur was built for him and there he worked for the last six years of his life. The word 'pasteurization' was coined from his name and perpetuates his memory. On his 70th birthday a public celebration was held for him at which the Quaker Lister addressed the Catholic Pasteur: 'Truly there does not exist in the wide world an individual to whom medical science owes more than to you.' Pasteur replied, 'The future will belong to those who have done most for suffering humanity. I refer to you my dear Lister.'

Following the important work of Pasteur in this field, the study of microorganisms was extensively advanced by several great German bacteriologists such as Robert Koch and Emil von Behring. Progress has continued right down to present time. The science of microbiology has thrown light on the cause of infections and contagious disease in all departments of medicine and surgery. Further reference will be made to some of these.

THE RELIEF OF PAIN

The growth of surgery had been restrained not only by what had seemed unavoidable sepsis, but by the acute pain suffered by the patient. It was therefore most opportune that a second liberation should have been developing alongside the first. The discovery of anaesthesia was one of the great events of the 19th century. The story begins with Thomas Beddoes, an eccentric late-18th century physician, who hoped to cure chest diseases by the inhalation of various gases, to which end he founded the Pneumatic Institution at Clifton, Bristol. His most important contribution, however, was to discover and foster the work of Humphry Davy. Sir Humphry Davy, as he was to become, was a Methodist and as a youth he had been apprenticed to a Penzance surgeon. In 1797, however, he decided to devote himself to chemistry. By 1800 he was experimenting on himself with nitrous oxide and foresaw that in future 'it may probably be used with advantage in surgical operations in which no great effusion of blood takes place'. Michael Faraday who succeeded Davy in the chair of chemistry at the Royal Institution, noted in 1815 that ether had similar properties to those of nitrous oxide. Ether thus became a possible alternative to nitrous oxide as an anaesthetic. Faraday was a member of a small Presbyterian sect known as Sandemanians, after Robert Sandeman the founder, and was proud of his eldership in their small church in London.

At a later date, in 1844 at Hartford, Connecticut, a dentist, Horace Wells, allowed himself to be anaesthetized by nitrous oxide for the extraction of a molar tooth, an operation which proved painless. But further unsatisfactory trials led to temporary abandonment of nitrous oxide and to the use of ether. The value of ether was demonstrated to surgeons in 1846 in Massachusetts Hospital by John Collins Warren. Another dentist William Morton, became interested in the use of ether and persuaded Warren to remove a vascular tumour of the lower jaw while he administered ether anaesthesia. An account of the favourable result was published in 1846. Subsequently Liston in London amputated a leg using ether anaesthesia, and continued to use this technique when he moved to Edinburgh.

In January 1847 James Young Simpson, then Professor of Obstetrics in Edinburgh, was the first to employ ether anaesthesia in midwifery. However, he soon came to realize the drawbacks of ether for this purpose. His attention was the drawn to chloroform. To test this before he used it in midwifery Simpson and some colleagues tried it on themselves as they sat around his dining room table inhaling the fumes of the evaporating fluid from a flask standing in warm water. Duncan Flockhart had supplied him with a sufficient quantity to do this.

Simpson had been appointed to the chair of obstetrics at Edinburgh at the young age of 29. He was an excellent teacher and had an ingenious mind. He introduced iron wire sutures (1858), the long obstetric forceps, acupressure (1860-1864) and many new methods in gynaecology and obstetrics such as the uterine sound (1843), the sponge tent, dilatation of the cervix uteri in diagnosis, and version in deformed pelves. His memoirs on fetal pathology and hermaphroditism are noteworthy. Historians of the 19th century seem to be agreed that he was 'one of the most remarkable personalities of his time'. Towards the end of his life when he was asked by a reporter what was his greatest discovery, he quietly replied: 'My greatest discovery was when I found that I was a sinner and that Jesus Christ was my Saviour.'

Since the late 19th century there has been much further progress in the discovery of new anaesthetics and safer techniques for their administration. Anaesthesia has become an important specialty. The anaesthetist has paved the way for the surgeon to perform skilled procedures in almost every part of the body in a way which in earlier centuries would have been quite inconceivable.

SAFER SURGERY – LISTER

The first of the British surgeons to grasp the full significance of Pasteur's discoveries and to apply them to surgery was Joseph Lister. His insight proved a turning point in history. Joseph Lister was born at Upton, Essex, into a Quaker family. His father was a successful wine merchant and an amateur microscopist who contributed to his hobby by inventing the achromatic lens. Joseph, the future Lord Lister, studied at University College Hospital, qualified in 1852, and then became house surgeon to James Syme in Edinburgh. Lister later married Syme's daughter Agnes and, in doing this, he 'married out' of the Society of Friends and joined his wife as a member of the Episcopal Church of Scotland. Agnes greatly encouraged him in his surgical work and it was a heavy blow to him when she died of pneumonia in Italy in 1893. In 1851 Lister occupied the Chair of Surgery in Glasgow and eighteen years later succeeded his previous chief Syme in the Chair of Surgery in Edinburgh. In 1877, however, he accepted the Chair of Surgery in King's College Hospital, London, in the hope that he could convince the London surgeons of the significance of his findings. He had given much thought to the problem of wound sepsis, especially during his time in Glasgow where he had conducted many careful experiments. When he read of the work of Pasteur and of the presence of microorganisms in the air and surroundings, he realized the relevance of this discovery to the problem of sepsis in the surgical wards. Then, reading of the use of carbolic acid in the sewers of Carlisle, he tried out the acid in surgery, originally using carbolic soaked dressings, but later also using his famous carbolic spray. The results were dramatic. He even opened a knee joint to wire a patella at which his contemporaries muttered 'malpraxis'. At first, most of the surgeons of his day were critical of his methods even though his former chief Syme was among the first to accept and use 'antiseptic surgery'. On the Continent, however, leading surgeons were at once interested and von Bergmann, while giving full credit to Lister, introduced steam sterilization (1886) and made his own techniques aseptic (1891). Eventually Lister lived to see his work acclaimed and in 1897 he was created a peer, the first medical man to receive this honour.

Lister's other contributions to medicine included the description (in 1852) of the muscles of the iris, studies of blood coagulation, the quest for absorbable sutures, the production of sterilized catgut and the introduction of gauze dressings. When Queen Victoria became concerned about his animal experiments and wrote to ask Lister to declare himself publicly against them, he explained to her that such experiments were being done to lessen human suffering.

The quiet spirit of his Quaker upbringing continued to guide him. Writing to his father about an important decision he wrote: 'It is true that it must entirely depend on myself (under the blessing, if I may humbly say so, of Almighty God in Jesus Christ) whether I succeed or not.' He was marked by an unusual courtesy, serenity and thoughtfulness for the patient. As Raymond Crawfurd, a physician of King's College Hospital has written, 'It was not the first time in the world's history that Providence, with purposeful wisdom, had chosen a man of superlative saintliness to be a medium of salvation to the world.'

AFTER LISTER

The history of surgery divides itself into 'before and after Lister'. His outlook and methods were speedily followed and improved upon in Germany, France and other countries of Europe and America, and numerous disciples themselves began to open new channels for an increasingly fruitful development of surgical techniques. For example, one of the most brilliant surgeons in Europe contemporary with Lister — Theodore Billroth, at Vienna — had been quick to accept and apply Listerian methods, as also had Karl Thiersch (pioneer in skin grafting), Richard Volkmann and Johann von Nussbaum. Nussbaum acted as communicator of their progress to Lister: 'Our results become better and better, the time of healing shorter, and pyaemia and erysipelas have completely disappeared.' Billroth went on to initiate many new operations and emerged as the virtual founder of abdominal surgery. He was the first to excise a cancer of the stomach and to complete a laryngectomy.

Two good examples of the work of active leading surgeons during the time of transition from the older to the newer surgery were James Syme of Edinburgh and James Paget of St. Bartholomew's Hospital, London.

In his own day James Syme was acknowledged as one of the ablest surgeons of Europe. Apart from a short, but not very happy, spell at University College Hospital, London, he spent the whole of his professional life in Edinburgh. He was a bold operator and showed that excision of joints was a feasible operation and could obviate amputation. He wrote a volume on his subject entitled *Excision of Diseased Joints* (1831). His name is familiar from the amputation through the ankle joint, which is still called after him. He published a volume on *Excision of Scapula* (1832) as well as a standard textbook of surgery entitled *Principles of Surgery* (1831). He was the first surgeon in Scotland to perform an amputation through the hip joint. He successfully treated an aneurysm of the iliac artery by ligating the artery above and below the aneurysm. He also excised a large sarcoma of the lower jaw. His mind was ever open to new progress and he was among the first to employ ether anaesthesia and to accept the work of his son-in-law, Lister. Dr. John Brown said of him that 'He never wasted a word, a drop of ink, or a drop of blood'. He was buried at St. John's Episcopal Church of which he had been a faithful member.

An older contemporary of Lister, James Paget, exercised a similar strong influence over the medical students and doctors in London. He was fundamentally a teacher and followed his students' later careers with interest. In an address on 'What becomes of medical students' he analysed, classified and discussed the careers of one thousand of his former students.

When he was a student in the anatomy room he had noted and recorded some small specks occurring in muscle tissue and demonstrated that they were in fact encysted worms of *Trichinella spiralis*. After qualifying, he spent some time as a teacher of anatomy and physiology at the Royal College of Surgeons and during this time he completed a catalogue of the specimens in the pathological museum. Among his clinical contributions were descriptions of the generalized bone disease osteitis deformans, also known as Paget's disease of bone, and a skin condition of the nipple which is always associated with carcinoma of the breast — Paget's disease of the nipple. Although not outstanding as an operator, he became a brilliant diagnostician so that the saying became popular: 'Go to Paget to find out what is wrong and then to Ferguson to have it cut out.' In spite of this he eventually built a very extensive practice. He was an eloquent speaker and published *Lectures on Surgical Pathology* (1853) and *Clinical Lectures and Essays* (1875).

In 1871 he was made a baronet and enjoyed a distinguished circle of friends. He is described as a man of 'deep religious conviction who never told a story or joke making jest of sacred words'. In later life, when they had moved house from St. Paul's to the West End, Sir James and Lady Paget are said to have walked every Sunday from Cavendish Square to the Cathedral to take part in worship. One of his sons became Bishop of Oxford, another Bishop of Chester and the third was the Stephen Paget who wrote *Confessio Medici*.

Following the widespread acceptance of Lister's methods there were advances in many countries in each department of surgery and some of the Continental and American research centres rose to international eminence. This was true of the new Johns Hopkins Hospital, Baltimore, which for some years became the leading American school for surgical progress, medical education and postgraduate research.

PROGRESS IN THE U.S.A.

The Johns Hopkins Hospital is a striking example of the impact of the Christian faith on Medicine both in its inauguration and in respect to some of its early staff. Johns Hopkins himself was born of Quaker parents and imbued with Quaker convictions. When their local Society decreed it, the members immediately freed all their slaves without compensation. Hopkins was a merchant, who had become wealthy by investing in the Baltimore and Ohio railroad. He gave the bulk of his fortune to the founding of a university and a hospital, both of which carry his name. In its first years the hospital was made famous by 'the Big Four': Welch, Halsted, Kelly and Osler, all of whom in boyhood and student days were in various ways influenced by the impact of active Christianity.

W. H. Welch was outstanding both as a pathologist and as the administrator chiefly responsible for much of the prestige and efficiency of the Medical School. For 34 years he was Professor of Pathology and among other advances, discovered the bacillus of gas gangrene. He was an excellent teacher and a man of wide culture. He eventually relinquished the chair of pathology and took up the chair of the history of medicine. The library at the Hopkins was erected in his honour as The Welch Memorial Library. Welch was brought up in a Christian family. Referring to his upbringing he wrote 'The religious faith which had come down from the New England fathers was still strong and life in the church was vigorous.' During his student days at Yale he also had some dramatic form of Christian experience, but in later days his Christian adherence seems somewhat to have lessened.

William Osler was of Canadian origin, the son of an Episcopal minister. He entered university in order to study for the ministry, but later changed to Medicine. Latterly his attitude to organized religion became more formal, but his extensive knowledge of the Bible never forsook him. The Christian ethic which he had earlier imbibed underlies all of his writings. In an address to Yale students on Sunday evening, April 20th, 1913 and published as *A Way of Life,* he said, 'Begin the day with Christ and His prayer — you need no other. Learn to know your Bible, though not perhaps as your fathers did. In forming character and shaping conduct its touch has still its ancient power.' He occupied the chair of Medicine at the Johns Hopkins Medical School and later became Regius Professor of Medicine at Oxford. His most significant work, published in 1898, was the *Principles and Practice of Medicine.* In 1898 he also founded the *Quarterly Journal of Medicine.* 'A master clinician, an inspiring teacher, a forceful speaker and a fascinating orator, he was a true leader of men. Endowed by nature with a charm of personality, buoyancy of spirit, a heart full of kindness and charity and a total stranger to envy and malice.' During his Oxford years he dominated the spirit of Medicine at that time.

Howard Kelly was the most consistently Christian figure of the four and throughout was outspoken in support of the faith. His main surgical interest was in gynaecology and Blair Bell claimed that he laid the foundations of scientific operative gynaecology. His consummate skill and the artistry of his operative technique made him easily the first among his fellow gynaecologists. He had already founded in 1883 and begun to develop the Kensington Hospital in Philadelphia. In 1888 he was appointed Professor of Gynaecology in the University of Pennsylvania but was pressed to transfer to the new Johns Hopkins a year later.

His contributions to medical science were many and varied. For example, he was a pioneer in the use of cocaine anaesthesia, he introduced the operations of suspension for retroversion of the uterus and of ureterectomy. He was among the first to practice aeroscopic examination of the bladder and catheterization of the ureters. He was also among the first to use wax-tipped bougies in the diagnosis of ureteric and renal calculi and to employ fluid injection to measure the pelvo-renal capacity in the diagnosis of hydronephrosis. He was early in the field of radium treatment of tumours and also suggested improvements in the operative techniques for vesico-vaginal fistula. Although the subsequent invention of X-rays rendered many of his investigations obsolete, their earlier significance for his day must not be overlooked. He produced two major works, *Operative Gynaecology* (1898) and *Medical Gynaecology* (1908), both illustrated by MacBrodel's celebrated drawings. These books included many of his own advances in gynaecology. His interests extended outside the field of Medicine and, with Burrage, he produced a *Dictionary of American Biography* (1928). Even late in life his mind continued to be active and together with Grant Ward he wrote a volume on *Electrosurgery* in 1932. The *Encyclopedia Americana* credits him with some five hundred articles in various journals.

Bernheim, one of the historians of the Johns Hopkins, wrote of him: 'He was the only surgeon I ever knew personally who indulged in prayer before he began operating. On the occasions I was present he called staff, nurses and visitors together in an anteroom and read a piece from the Bible or gave a prayer. A brief sincere gesture that you could see came from the man's innermost being.' He venerated the Bible and stoutly defended it. 'Few of my scientific friends,' he said, 'are aware that their science flourishes best in a land where the Bible is honoured. Where the Bible is dishonoured life becomes cheap and science an early victim.' He expressed his faith both in words and in deed. He worked enthusiastically in philanthropic projects, Christian teaching and downtown rescue work. He constantly affirmed that his Christian faith inspired a deeper interest in, and tenderness for, all men.

The surgical member of the 'Big Four' at the Hopkins was William S. Halsted, the professor of surgery. He proved a brilliant operator and the list of the new operations which he was the first to attempt is a long one. He was a pioneer in the use of infiltration anaesthesia with cocaine. He also carried asepsis to new standards by the use of gutta-percha tissues for drainage, rubber gloves in the operating theatre, silver foil dressings and much else of assistance in the finer operating techniques. He was also unequalled in his day as a trainer of postgraduates in the art and practice of surgery. Educated under Christian influences he, in contrast with his friend Howard Kelly, always remained very reserved in expressing spiritual matters.

William Keen performed the first successful operation in the United States for a brain tumour. He had been one of the first American surgeons to adopt the Listerian technique. Indeed, prior to Lister, to attempt to remove a cranial tumour would have been criminal folly. The operation was done in 1887 and the patient lived for some 30 years.

Keen became Professor of Surgery at Jefferson Medical College. He wrote an eight volume *System of Surgery*. He was also the author of an important work on the surgical complications and sequels of typhoid fever. He was very popular as a lecturer and teacher and addressed both the American Medical Association and the Royal College of Surgeons of England. A Baptist and an accomplished preacher, he spoke frequently for different Christian causes and wrote several Christian publications. A man of deep humility, he expressed his faith in such remarks as 'Surely our hearts should be lifted in gratitude to God for giving us such splendid powers of reasoning, experiment and research, all for the service of our fellow men'.

Oliver Wendel Holmes was another son of the manse. Originally he opted for Law, but later switched to Medicine. He studied at Harvard where, after practising in Boston, he became Professor of Anatomy and Physiology in 1847. He is chiefly known for his literary work, in particular for *The Autocrat, The Professor* and *The Poet at the Breakfast Table.* He coined the word 'anaesthesia' and produced a paper on the *Contagiousness of Puerperal Fever,* published in 1843. The *Encyclopedia Americana* describes this paper as the first important contribution to medical research by an American physician. Holmes had been brought up in an extreme Calvinistic background against which he reacted strongly, becoming a Unitarian. One of his poems 'Lord of all being throned afar', is included in many of the Church hymnaries. It ends with the couplet 'Grant us Thy truth to make us free, and kindling hearts that burn for Thee'.

According to the historian Douglas Guthrie, the most picturesque figure in American Medicine was Daniel Drake. He was the first after Hippocrates and Sydenham to give attention to geographical pathology and he made several contributions to the topography of disease. He has left a description of his boyhood in *Pioneer Life in Kentucky.* Born in poverty among the log cabins of Kentucky, he achieved his education by determined self-help and eventually graduated at the Philadelphia medical college. He then travelled widely and, in course of time, founded medical schools at Ohio and Cincinatti. He became editor of *The Western Journal of Medical Science* and completed *The Principal Diseases of the Interior Valley of North America* in two volumes. His various travels had made him acquainted with the geographical distribution of diseases, especially of fevers, in the various parts of the Mississippi valley. He originated from a long line of Baptist pioneers. After his marriage, however, his wife helped to organize the first Episcopal Church in Cincinatti which he joined, but he also organized a society to perpetuate the simple faith of his parents.

Ephraim McDowell was a pioneer of abdominal surgery, successfully performing oöphorectomy for ovarian cyst. This, his first operation, was performed in December 1809 long before the Listerian methods came into use. It was entirely successful and on the fifth day his patient was up making her own bed, and by the twenty-fifth day she had returned to her own home some sixty miles away, where she lived for a further 32 years. Altogether McDowell performed 13 oöphorectomies and eight of the patients lived. In the context of the appalling mortality from any operation in the early 19th century this was no mean accomplishment. He also performed 22 lithotomies without any mortality. He had learned his surgical technique from John Bell of Edinburgh where many Americans came to study Medicine in the 18th and early 19th centuries. McDowell came from a Presbyterian family and his father was a lawyer, who eventually became a judge. His wife was an Episcopalian and it is said that after his marriage he gave up 'stern Presbyterianism for the gentler faith'.

The road to safer surgery was not achieved by giants alone. Many lesser men contributed discovery, suggestion and example. There were other factors. Urgent needs in two world wars and the practical exigencies of polar expeditions speeded the solution of vital problems which might otherwise have lagged. In the history of surgery there is yet another debt. A high price, at the outset, was paid by the early radiologists. A tribute to their memory will be in place.

When Wilhelm Konrad von Roentgen in 1896 and Pierre and Marie Curie in 1898 respectively reported on the value of X-rays and radium, few realized the dangers of the processes which they were handling. Until the staffs of radiology departments were properly protected, many of the workers contracted various forms of malignancy. It was another example of martyrdom in the cause of Science and Medicine. It is good to be able to add that recent therapeutic success indicates that those sacrifices were not in vain. We must, however, never forget the price at which many successful branches of modern medicine have been bought.

CHAPTER 8

PIONEERS IN PREVENTIVE MEDICINE

PREVENTIVE medicine and immunology in their full scientific applications could not develop until after the basic discoveries in microbiology of Pasteur, Virchow, Koch and other pioneers of the 19th century. Hence the history of preventive medicine falls into two eras, before and after Pasteur, and it is the later era that contains most of the story. This does not mean, however, that a number of facts of public health were not known or that preventive medicine was not practised empirically in the earlier centuries — as we have already seen. A brief summary must here suffice.

THE DARK AND MIDDLE AGES

With the Fall of Rome many of the beginnings of public health were lost. These included personal hygiene as practised by the Greek athletes and public hygiene as exemplified by aqueducts (for pure water supplies), public baths and latrines of the Romans. As morals deteriorated and sexual promiscuity increased, the practice of mixed bathing led to the contamination of the public facilities. The baths later became centres of the prolific spread of disease.

One reaction on the part of Christians was mistaken and unfortunate. There was a move towards asceticism, that is, the neglect of the needs of the body in pursuit of a better spiritual life. But not all sections of the Church were influenced in this direction. In Asia Minor there remained 'the light in the East'. The Byzantine Empire and the Christian communities retained much of Graeco-Roman Medicine and Hygiene. Similarly the newer monasteries tended to set an example by the quality of their buildings, good water supply and drainage. The siting of monasteries at the junction of the main travel routes offered facilities to travellers and those who were sick. They must indirectly have contributed to public health by example.

During the Middle Ages the monks offered a rudimentary first-aid service to the wounded men from the Crusades and other armies on the march. There were, too, the beginnings of 'quarantine' (derived from the prescription of '40 days' of isolation). The sufferers from leprosy were also segregated into the lazar houses (p. 13).

One of the chief centres from which came progress in the teaching of preventive medicine was the School of Salerno (p. 37). It was one of the first medical schools to call for a recognized qualification for those who wished to practise Medicine. It was also the earliest of the medical centres to think in terms of medical education and an agreed curriculum. But perhaps its chief wider influence on Europe was through the long poem *Regimen Sanitatis Salernitanum* (The Code of Health of the School of Salerno). This book was a series of health rules in some (originally) 362 verses. It is said, however, to have grown steadily in the course of its many editions to over 3500 verses! It is certain that it was the most popular medieval book, carrying its jingles through the centuries until Renaissance times.

EARLY LEADERS

A number of individual doctors stood out as early pioneers in preventive medicine. In the 16th century Girolamo Fracastoro (p. 55) clearly advocated measures for public health, particularly in his book *De Contagione (Concerning Contagion)*. He was the first to present a consistent theory of contagion and to recognize the communicable nature of several diseases such as typhus and tuberculosis. Similarly, Guillaume de Baillou, Dean of the Medical Faculty in Paris, accurately described the nature of whooping cough, diphtheria, plague and rheumatism.

It is in the 18th century that welcome and long overdue steps began to be taken in the interests of the health of children. Thomas Coram's care of the foundlings (p. 24) was followed by a leading London physician's plea for a thorough approach to the diseases and preventive medicine of childhood. William Cadogan, in his *Essay upon Nursing* (1748), strongly advocated breast feeding and sought to bring to an end a number of unhelpful and debilitating customs in the rearing of children. He went on to outline a number of basic rules that were desirable in the pursuit of child health.

18TH CENTURY PUBLIC HEALTH

Some of the most effective steps in preventive medicine which were taken in the 18th century were the results of new social interest springing up in the more progressive Christian communities – the Puritans of New England and the Methodists and the Quakers in England. In these communities there were frequent instances of the advocacy of health measures by an enlightened minister, and the effects on the general public of an example given by his congregation.

The robust mind of the Puritan preacher Cotton Mather in Boston became concerned for the general health of his congregation. After investigating a virulent measles epidemic in the area, he turned to smallpox which, he noted, frequently spread from around the port. Mather was a corresponding member of the Royal Society and had learnt of the beginnings of inoculation from its circulated papers. He discussed it with the local authorities and (though not supported by the doctors) he eventually became one of the first writers to put forward in his animalcular theses a basically correct theory of immunology. Having first advocated it to his church (with a lukewarm medical support) he persuaded the public authorities to be prepared to make a trial of inoculation when the next smallpox epidemic occurred. In one series 242 persons were inoculated and of these only six died. The mortality rate was 2.5% as compared with 15% in the corresponding group of the uninoculated. While the early methods of inoculation still carried grave risks and there was still very much to be learned, Cotton Mather truly deserves to be ranked as a significant pioneer in American preventive medicine.

A large place of influence in the growth of public health in England was occupied by the evangelist John Wesley. The zeal and industry of this truly remarkable figure are beyond praise. It is believed that he travelled on his faithful horses over a quarter of a million miles and preached over 40,000 sermons in the villages and cities – not to speak of the work involved in publishing a whole series of the literary classics to educate his local preachers. Among these books was his own *Primitive Physick: or an Easy and Natural Method of Curing Most Diseases* (1747). It was a home medical guide from which the local preachers were encouraged to give guidance to the Methodist people. While it contains references to some of the mistakes of folk medicine and to some of the useless nostrums of the age, on the whole it provides much common sense and sound practical advice for personal hygiene. Like the Puritans, Wesley was fond of soap and water. It is from this book that has come the phrase 'Cleanliness is, indeed, next to Godliness'. The advice came to exercise a general salutary influence upon the nation's health.

Circulating at the same time as Wesley's *Primitive Physic* was a similar volume by a Scotsman — William Buchan's *Domestic Medicine or the Family Physician.* Both volumes went through many editions. Buchan began at Edinburgh University as a theological student but changed to the medical faculty.

JOHN HOWARD AND PRISONS

From the first, the Religious Society of Friends (Quakers) were interested in such matters as personal hygiene and public health. Again and again a Quaker physician or layman is found in the vanguard of groups of public-spirited men intent on social and health reforms. Some, such as Lettsom, have already been mentioned in earlier chapters, but reference should be made to one of the greatest of their pioneers, Howard.

The reforms of John Howard applied to the management of the prisons, hospitals and lazarettos of Europe had much to do with the suppression of typhus fever. In his position as High Sheriff of Bedfordshire, Howard had seen some of the appallingly filthy conditions and iniquities of the prison system in which unpaid gaolers depended on what they could extract from the prisoners or their friends. Moreover he himself had seen the inside of prisons when a ship in which he was sailing was captured by French privateers and he had been kept in prison. The experience led him subsequently to make extensive journeys throughout England and Europe inspecting gaols and lazarettos. As a result of his report on the *State of the Prisons in England and Wales* he succeeded in getting two Acts of Parliament passed (1774) which did much to relieve the position. He emphasized the need for a paid prison staff, simple hygienic measures — including the baking of the clothes of prisoners — and avoidance of overcrowding. By such measures the incidence of gaol fever (typhus) was greatly reduced, not only in the prisons but also in the navy which employed numbers of ex-prisoners who constantly carried the infection with them from prison to naval quarters.

Later he was invited to inspect and to comment also on the hospitals. Although not medically qualified, he attended the sick poor and those in need. Travelling in winter in Russia he was asked to call to see an English lady with a febrile illness. He himself contracted the fever and died of it. He was a man of deeply religious feeling. It is said of him that 'his evangelical opinions were intense, but he was free from religious bigotry'.

THE BEGINNINGS OF IMMUNOLOGY

Perhaps the most far-reaching single advance in preventive medicine during the 18th century was Jenner's discovery that smallpox could be prevented by vaccination. By its use smallpox has today been eradicated throughout the world.

Edward Jenner had been a pupil of John Hunter and maintained a close correspondence with him after he had returned to practise in Berkeley in his native Gloucestershire. Jenner was not the first to vaccinate a person with cowpox to protect him from smallpox. Benjamin Jesty, a Dorsetshire farmer, having observed that cowpox protected against a subsequent attack of smallpox, vaccinated his wife with material from the vesicles of cowpox when an outbreak of smallpox occurred in his village. Although she survived, she had a severe febrile reaction and this, together with the adverse criticism from the villagers, discouraged Jesty so much that he did not repeat the experiment. On the Continent Peter Platt reported to Kiel University that he had successfully vaccinated a number of children, while a Protestant pastor in France stated that cowpox vaccination was as effective as arm to arm inoculation and was much safer.

Jenner, however, was the first to study carefully the procedure and to publicize it among the members of the medical profession. To demonstrate its efficiency he vaccinated a boy, James Phipps, and when he subsequently inoculated him with material from a smallpox lesion he demonstrated that the boy was immune to the disease. He published the results of his findings and experiments in 1798. This is one of the significant dates in the history of Medicine. In subsequent papers Jenner discussed the complications of vaccination. The practice rapidly became accepted, and in *The Medical and Physical Journal* for 1801 it is described as 'this happy discovery (which) in less than three years has been communicated to every enlightened people, even the remotest in the world'. In the same volume a Dr. Clement confesses that he was sceptical of vaccination at first, but by the beginning of the year he had vaccinated nearly two hundred persons and was satisfied with its safety and efficacy.

Jenner was the son of a country clergyman and his wife was also a vicar's daughter. She was a woman of deep piety which expressed itself in practical ways such as founding a Sunday School for the village children. His eldest brother Stephen also entered the ministry. It is not surprising that Jenner should have acquired a strong Christian faith. Throughout his lifetime he refused invitations to assume more prestigious posts and continued to serve his Gloucestershire villagers, the poor of whom he vaccinated free of charge.

Over the same periods of the 18th century came advances in other directions, such as the discovery of deficiency diseases caused by defective diets. One of the most beneficial of these was the work of James Lind, an Edinburgh medical graduate who entered the Naval Medical Service and published in 1753 his *Treatise on Scurvy*. A century and a half before vitamin C was discovered, Lind had shown that fresh fruit, vegetables, and especially oranges and lemons (which contained the vitamin) had reduced the incidence of, or eliminated, scurvy from the ships' crews on long voyages. When it was found possible to preserve and store the juices of the citrus fruits, prophylaxis against the distressing and deady 'scourge of the sea' was completed.

Lind followed up his work on scurvy with other observations and in 1757 published *Most Effectual Means of Preserving the Health of Seamen*. He also made a study of typhus fever and recommended thorough delousing measures such as bathing, a change into clean clothes and baking the lice-infected garments. Lind's work had a far-reaching effect in both the Navy and Army. Little of Lind's personal biography has survived, but at each point where a glimpse is allowed, he comes over as an utterly admirable character, not unlike Jenner. He was loyal, industrious, unassuming and had a great sense of duty. When settled as the physician at the Naval Hospital he seems not to have resented the fact that his serving colleagues in high places, who had all made use of his findings, were given many honours while he received none. After his death the only tribute was a memorial tablet on the walls of the Church which he and his widow attended in his retirement. It is still there, in St. Mary's, Portchester, and all it adds to the factual details is, 'James Lind, M.D., who was for twenty-five years Physician of the Royal Hospital at Haslar'.

EVANGELICAL REFORMERS

Shaftesbury was the leader of the second generation of the Evangelical Party in the Church of England, which, led by Wilberforce, had been responsible for the abolition of the slave trade in 1807. Shaftesbury entered Parliament in 1826 and was actually engaged in religious and social reform for the rest of his life. Not without much difficulty and opposition he at last brought through Parliament a series of beneficent measures, which regulated the hours and conditions of work. The Mines Act 1842 prohibited employment of women and girls in mines and collieries and reduced hours for boys; the Ten Hours Factory Act 1847 controlled the hours for women and children in the textile factories; the Common Lodging Houses Act 1851 required the maintenance of certain standards.

Shaftesbury went on to interest himself in housing, education (including 'Ragged Schools') and many aspects of social need. A considerable number of these had influence on health. Throughout his long and honourable life much of what he took up worked in the direction of public health.

While Shaftesbury worked from the upper crust of society downwards, the first general of the Salvation Army, William Booth, spread his influence from the bottom upwards. In the first instance Booth did not set out to be a social or medical reformer. He knew very well that 'you cannot make a man clean by washing his shirt'. His aim was purely spiritual and he 'saved the people in battalions'. But he had a deep love and interest in them and when their souls were right he wanted everything else to be right including their environment. As a result, all over the world the Salvation Army has been outstanding in its social and medical services at points of special need (pp. 147, 158). Both directly and indirectly it has contributed to the world need of preventive medicine.

Many similar benefactors of mankind in other branches of preventive medicine and immunology are mentioned in other chapters — as, for example, in tropical medicine (p. 159). Both among the armed services and government services of various colonial powers of the 19th century, and among the missionaries from Europe and America, Christian doctors have been household names. Many have shown commendable heroism and persistence under the most daunting circumstances in their quest for the secret of a prevailing tropical disease. One who caught the public attention of the U.S.A. in 1900 was Walter Reed, who led the courageous group which served the American Yellow Fever Commission by going to Havana to study an outbreak in the U.S. army (see p. 161).

MODERN DEVELOPMENTS

From the time when, through the work of Pasteur, Virchow, Koch and others, the nature of infection by microorganisms had become fully understood, various preventive measures have been applied to successive areas of need. Towards the end of the 19th century the pace quickened.

The lone pioneer, often pursuing his quest against the scepticism of medical colleagues and the hostility of the public, has been replaced by highly organized departments of technical research. The individual worker now usually shares success with a highly trained team.

The factors which have brought the most effective and widespread beneficial results in national health have been the enactments of central and local governments to enforce proper standards in plumbing, water supplies, milk supplies, sewage disposal, reduction of air pollution and all the other contributing measures of preventive medicine. The various Public Health Acts and the recommendations of various Commissions have in the long run saved more lives than all the curative drugs in the pharmacopoeia.

There is still a large place for the medical profession in public health. But training members of the public in the principles of preventive medicine and successfully persuading them fully to apply the principles is still of the highest priority. In this operation Christians have played, and are still playing, a useful part, for example, by the self-discipline which helps to reduce excessive drinking, smoking and other contemporary health hazards. Judging by statistics published from time to time, there is a new need and a new challenge to the Churches and to individual Christians again to exercise their influence in these and similar directions.

In many parts of the world today where the first health priority is for wells to be bored, latrines to be dug and other elements of public health to be applied, most of the Christian missions are able to offer first aid in these respects and in health education, while awaiting government or W.H.O. projects. There must still be a big place for curative measures, but the future of health lies with preventive medicine.

HISTORICAL MISREPRESENTATION

Several of the general books of the history of Medicine, and some sectional studies have stated or implied that some of the main lines of advance have been collectively opposed by religious circles. A false picture has been given. In June 1977 Alfred D. Fair submitted a Ph.D. thesis to the Open University under the title *Medical Developments and Religious Belief, with Special Reference to the 18th and 19th Centuries.* The following is a summary of his findings.

He selected three areas where it has been alleged that scientific medicine and religion had reacted in conflict —

1. *Inoculation for Smallpox* (about 1720): He found that a few local and

scattered Calvinist communities in Scotland had raised objections, but mainly against compulsion. The objections did not recur on the introduction of Jenner's cowpox vaccination in 1798 and were not heard in the 19th century. J. W. Draper's statement (1875) that the clergy 'strenuously resisted' inoculation and A. D. White's echo (1895) of 'bitter denunciation of inoculation by the English clergy' appear to be pure historical artefacts.

2. *Anaesthesia:* It is often said that the use of anaesthesia in obstetrics was met by 'massive religious opposition' when introduced in 1847. Evidence for any such state of affairs appears to be virtually non-existent. The 'conflict' seems to be a myth, based on a defence prepared in advance by James Young Simpson himself against an attack which never materialized! Search among the copies of contemporary newspapers and the religious press gives no support for any such 'conflict'.

3. *Unborn Children:* There have certainly been debates lasting from the 19th century and up to the present time concerning the status of unborn children in any consideration of the problems of abortion, embryotomy and Caesarean section. But apart from debate raised by the Roman Catholic Church's placing an absolute value on fetal life, mass religious opposition has been absent. On the contrary, there is no evidence for an overall 'warfare' between religion and Medicine, nor for opposition to orthodox scientific Medicine by the established churches of England and Scotland, or the nonconformist bodies in England and America.

CHAPTER 9

MEDICAL EDUCATION AND
MEDICAL STUDENTS

IT was not until the mid-19th century that a comprehensive medical curriculum was fully established in the medical colleges of the United Kingdom. In earlier centuries there had been small medieval schools of medicine, several medical corporations and royal colleges had been founded, and prominent physicians and surgeons had operated an apprentice system. On the Continent of Europe somewhat fuller provisions had already been made in most countries before the crucial Medical Act of 1858 at last created the General Medical Council of Great Britain and Ireland. This body had the effect not only of rationalizing the somewhat piecemeal requirements of the various medical corporations and moving towards more generally acceptable standards, but also of unifying the profession.

Reference has already been made, especially in Chapter 2, to some of the earliest rudimentary forms of medical training. Some of the first Christian hospitals in early centuries welcomed medical students and deaconesses for such knowledge of medical treatment and nursing as they had to share. Several institutions in the Near East gained an early international reputation. This became even more true of the chief monastic hospitals, as, for example, Monte Cassino in Southern Italy. Charlemagne and Alfred the Great are recorded as having legislated in their domains for choir schools to be attached to each of the cathedrals, which were also to help educate additional pupils. It was proposed that suitable boys should be selected and encouraged to take up Medicine as their chief interest and vocation. During the Middle Ages, on a wide scale, the monastic infirmaries regularly played their part in the training of priest-doctors.

THE UNIVERSITIES

It was, however, as a result of the rise of the universities across Europe that the more formal and academic side of medical training began to grow. Between the years 1100 and 1500, while the Church's interests were mainly ecclesiastical and theological, the majority of the new university foundations came to have their own medical faculties. Their teachers and libraries attracted students and they began to play an increasingly international role. This became especially true of Salerno, Montpellier, Bologna, Padua and Paris.

There was, however, a price to be paid for the new standards of lecturing and demonstrating, especially in anatomy at a time when dissection of the human body was not permitted. The effect was to accentuate the theoretical content of all lecturing and for those being trained to be moved further away from clinical observation of the patient and his disease. In earlier centuries, since the teaching of Galen, as compared with others, was thought to be not inconsistent with the Christian faith, the Church authorities had authorized the study of his works. Because of the virtual infallibility which Galen acquired, it was not possible to correct the anatomical errors derived from his dissections of animals. The updating of anatomy had to await the impact of the Renaissance.

Of the first universities and colleges the most immediately interesting was the Medical School at Salerno, which in effect was a single medical faculty attaining university standards. It was unique in that, during the 200 years of its special prominence as a teaching centre, it enjoyed considerable liberty from the ecclesiastical authorities in spite of – or perhaps because of – the proximity of the great Monte Cassino monastery. It further had a number of laymen as teachers instead of all monks. It also had a cosmopolitan staff which resembled those of a present-day hospital situated in a multiracial and multireligious area in which the various traditions have agreed to cooperate medically for the common good. Salerno was early the site of a bishopric and later an archbishopric. It had a Benedictine cloister and hospital as early as 820, probably pioneered from Monte Cassino. After the Norman conquest of Italy the different racial elements in Southern Italy were welded together by the Normans, and the medical school seems to have settled for what was best from the four traditions of Greek, Latin, Hebrew and Arabic, of which the Greek tradition came through from Christian sources such as Monte Cassino. After some 200 years other universities took its place, but it did not finally close until 1811 by order of Napoleon.

In its first period of prosperity Salerno gained much from the arrival, as foreign secretary to the Duke of Apulia, of a Christian known as Constantine the African. Not long after his arrival he became a monk at Monte Cassino and spent the rest of his life translating into Latin the

Arab manuscripts, which he had obtained in North Africa. Monte Cassino was also one of the centres concerned with circulating other medical manuscripts. The physicians of Salerno themselves continued to publish many books, including a complete encyclopaedia of Medicine to which all the staff had contributed. The organization and spirit of Salerno, with due status for its teachers, the systematic lecturing, and the desire not to miss any new knowledge, had communicated itself to other universities such as Bologna and Padua before the Renaissance.

Another progressive university centre was Montpellier. Founded about 738, there are records of visits by the Archbishop of Mainz in 1137 in order 'to listen to medical lectures' and later St. Bernard describes a similar visit in 1153 by the Archbishop of Lyons. In 1181 the Count of Mountpellier declared it a 'free medical school'. (The University of Montpellier had been founded in 1180.) Among its stronger points was its readiness to welcome real progress from whatever quarter it came.

Montpellier was the second main place of entry for Arabic medical literature from North Africa and Spain, the latter also being a translation centre. It was famous, however, as a postgraduate medical training school to which a number of the leading French physicians and surgeons went and others from the international ranks, including some from the British Isles. In later times, as during the troublous years of the religious wars, Montpellier tended to adhere to an independent and progressive course.

Until the early 19th century Oxford and Cambridge remained the only two universities in England at which Medicine could be studied. A number of their graduates, whenever the cost could be met, opted to transfer for postgraduate study in Montpellier, Paris, Bologna or Padua. There were not wanting, however, patriotic physicians who sought to encourage appropriate facilities in England. This became especially true when the effects of Renaissance had become widespread. One such benefactor was Thomas Linacre, a Fellow of All Souls, an accomplished Greek scholar and sympathetic to the 'new learning' and Reformation. He sought to restore a clearer appreciation of the scientific outlook of the Greeks and to reinstate observation and experiment. As one means to this end in 1524 he endowed a lectureship designed to apply the 'new learning' both at Oxford and Cambridge. In a number of other ways Linacre sought to promote progress.

Another of the benefactors was the celebrated physician and high Churchman, John Caius who sought specially to benefit Gonville College, Cambridge. He so disposed of his wealth that it would enable the university authorities to refound and rebuild the college under the name of Gonville and Caius College. In addition he established at the College a number of medical fellowships for postgraduate students and in other ways endeavoured to promote Medicine. He also remembered the needs of the anatomy department by obtaining from the judicial authorities an annual grant to the College of two corpses of executed criminals for dissection.

Other philanthropists have from time to time made further generous bequests, for example, at the suggestion of his friend Richard Mead, John Radcliffe left two postgraduate fellowships to the Medical Faculty in Oxford. They were to be tenable for ten years, five of which were available for study in an overseas university.

SCOTLAND

The Scottish Universities were founded in the 15th and 16th centuries – St. Andrew's (1411), Glasgow (1451), Aberdeen (1494) and Edinburgh's 'Town College' (1583). While Aberdeen was the first to appoint a medical member of staff, the Scottish universities for some years did not award a medical degree. John Knox, in the Book of Discipline, proposed that St. Andrew's should have a medical faculty, but with its small population, and very few local practising physicians, little came of this.

Scottish doctors at that time crossed to France for further study and qualification. After the Civil War they went to the reformed University of Leyden, which had been founded by William the Silent as a reward to the people of the city for their resistance in the siege. At the height of his prominence at Leyden as Professor of Medicine, Boerhaave attracted many from the British Isles – Scottish and English nonconformists – to this university. Its influence was to promote the virtual refounding of the faculty in Edinburgh, which proved subsequently of great advantage to the Quakers and other nonconformists (excluded from Oxford and Cambridge) who came there. Most of those coming from the American colonies to qualify in Britain also benefited.

THE ROYAL COLLEGES

By the 16th century there was a marked trend for the various types of practitioner to come together into corporations. In the capital cities the physicians, the surgeons and the apothecaries (the general practitioners of their times) began to associate for the purposes of licensing and the regulation of professional work. Though much of their work was concerned with licenses to practice and remuneration, some measures were adopted to ensure more regularized standards in day-to-day practice.

In London, Thomas Linacre, physician both to Henry VII and Henry VIII, endeavoured successfully to interest the King in the work of physicians. Henry, in 1518, granted a charter to establish the Royal College of Physicians of London, making Linacre the first President. Linacre's house also became its first official building. It was not, however, until 1540 that Henry VIII granted a special charter for the Barber-Surgeons, a body which later, in 1745, became known as the Company of Surgeons and in 1800 as the Royal College of Surgeons. With a number of difficulties arising from relationships with the City Companies of London, the Worshipful Society of Apothecaries — who were the general practitioners of the day — was not incorporated until 1617.

Scotland offers an interesting picture associated with the provisions for Glasgow. Before the Royal College of Physicians of Edinburgh (1681) and Royal College of Surgeons of Edinburgh (1778) had been founded, the West of Scotland had from 1599 had its Faculty of Physicians and Surgeons of Glasgow. (In recent years it has changed its title to the Royal College of Physicians and Surgeons of Glasgow.) The Faculty originated with Peter Lowe, a Scot who, after having been trained in Orleans and at St. Côme in Paris, became a Major-Surgeon with the Spanish armies and then, on changing to the Protestant side, Major-Surgeon with the armies of Henry of Navarre. On returning to Scotland he gave much of his attention to the local needs for due standards of medical care to be ensured on the Western side of Scotland. He was appointed by James VI to survey the position and to test the validity and competence of those professing to practise medicine or surgery. In the event the various measures adopted for due licensing of those entering practice led to the organization of the Faculty as the administrative authority for standards. Possibly influenced by some of the prominent French physicians and surgeons who had long advocated it, Lowe strongly urged the desirability of the various branches of the medical profession remaining together. They did this in Glasgow and have continued to do so to the present.

THE RESULTING CURRICULUM

It is not the intention here to trace in detail the evolution of modern medical training. Like so much else in Medicine it was a long time in coming and there remains room for improvement. The German medical historian, T. Puschman, once commented: 'The customs of the Middle Ages in regard to medical teaching have been preserved longest in England!' He did concede, however, that the lecturers in science departments sought to communicate a truly scientific attitude, and he was duly impressed by the comprehensive Public Health Act of 1875 and its applications in all aspects of Medicine. Much recent progress in the planning of the curriculum has been made.

It was a turning point for Britain when the Medical Act of 1858 appointed the General Medical Council for Medical Education and Registration. Its primary duty was to ensure that only the names of adequately trained and otherwise fit medical trainees should be placed on the official register of medical practitioners and, for sufficient cause, to remove the names of any who may have become unworthy. In the course of its work two other important duties have devolved upon it – (i) inspection of the training curriculum, teaching standards and examinations of the Medical Faculties and Colleges; and (ii) continual scrutiny of the drugs included in the British Pharmacopoeia. Today much time and care is bestowed by responsible and highly trained persons to ensure the preservation of the best standards in practice.

There have been many Christians among the public spirited men who have given much of their time to these necessary duties. Prominent among them was Charles Hastings, the sixth son of the Vicar of Martley, Worcestershire. Hastings was taught by two surgeons at Stourport and in London for a few months by four physicians and surgeons, after the fashion of the day. After what to us today seems a far too short apprenticeship he returned to Worcester in 1812 to be a house surgeon at the County Infirmary. He was then only eighteen! Later he went for three years to Edinburgh where he graduated M.D. On his return he was appointed a physician of the Worcester County Infirmary and became the leading practitioner of the city.

Hastings' whole professional life was devoted to efforts to raise the standard of provincial medical practice in the pursuit of which he founded a medical journal and in 1832, the Provincial Medical and Surgical Association. The latter was eventually merged into the national organization which in 1856 took the name British Medical Association. The major aim of Hastings and many others was to secure the comprehensive legislation of the 1858 Medical Act which would unite the profession and enforce due standards. He undertook his immense load of voluntary administrative work with a true sense of vocation. From his comments when, during the last B.M.A. meeting which he attended, he led the B.M.A. members into the special service in King's College, Cambridge, it was consciously his Nunc Dimittis.

WOMEN DOCTORS

Although it may not be obvious from the usual silence in modern biography on spiritual matters, there was a strong Christian element in the motivation of the pioneers of medical education for women. The first stirrings came from Elizabeth Blackwell and she made it something of a moral crusade. She was the daughter of a Bristol sugar refiner, who was a Dissenter and active reformer. When her family went to the U.S.A. and came on more difficult times, she supported herself by teaching while trying to study anatomy with the help of doctor friends. Eventually she was able to register for a medical course in Geneva University, N.Y. State, and took her M.D. degree in 1849 with honours. After many disappointments, backed by a group of women Quakers, she set up a dispensary for women and children in a depressed district of New York. She later established in New York a hospital and medical school for women.

The next move was in England by Elizabeth Garrett, daughter of an Aldeburgh business man. Her family was devout and she was influenced by philanthropic motives. Through a school friend she met Emily Davies, daughter of the Rector of Gateshead, and became interested in the Langham Place Group, a circle of West End ladies interested in social reform. She was encouraged in her aim to study medicine by Emily Davies, Mrs Russell Gurney and others of the Group; and also by Dr Blackwell who happened to be in London on a visit. Her efforts to get into any of the medical faculties were disappointed. So she took private tuition and eventually qualified in 1865 by means of the Licentiate of the Society of Apothecaries, through which her name was placed on a medical register. Later she obtained her M.D. from Paris.

Another pioneer was Ann E. Clark. When she failed to gain acceptance at Edinburgh she went to study in Berne, and then returned to take her M.R.C.P. at Dublin. After several postgraduate studies abroad, she was appointed Surgeon to the Women's Hospital and the Children's Hospital in Birmingham. She was associated with Lawson Tait who at that time was developing his pioneer work in abdominal surgery and especially his operation for removing ovarian cysts. Ann Clark's religious motivation is clear from her lifelong membership of, and regular attendance at, the Bull Street meetings of the Quakers.

It was some years before more than a handful of women could get their names on the register and Sophia Jex-Blake had a particularly hard fight. She, too, came from a deeply religious family and received support from circles of Christian women. After applying to several universities, she was allowed (with several other women) to matriculate and study at Edinburgh, but not to take the degree examination and qualify. She went to Berne and obtained the M.D. from there and then finally qualified for a place on the British register with the M.R.C.P. of Dublin in 1877. With the support of Elizabeth Garrett Anderson, Sophia Jex-Blake went on to found and to gain official recognition for the London School of Medicine for Women, with clinical teaching facilities at the Royal Free Hospital.

The first woman doctor to go overseas to bring Western Medicine to the women of Asia was an American, Clara Swain. She began work in 1869 under the auspices of the Board of Missions of the Methodist Church. By 1874 she had built the Clara Swain Hospital on a site donated by the Nawab of Rampur at Bareilly. Within ten years she had treated over 7000 women patients and received a royal welcome when called by the Rajah of Rajputana to attend his seriously ill wife. Her example was followed by a long line of women doctors dedicated to the women and children of India. Many of these were trained at the London School of Medicine for Women and the Royal Free Hospital (see p. 168).

Eventually there emerged from the countries of Asia women doctors from among their own peoples. Outstanding amongst them was Dr Hilda Lazarus. She came from a third generation Christian family, whose members had already given distinguished service in various other spheres. Qualifying from Madras Medical College, she came to Scotland and England for postgraduate study in obstetrics and gynaecology, obtaining the F.R.C.S. of Edinburgh. In later years in appreciation of her great work she received many honorary degrees and medals. She served successively as Superintendent of the Purdah Hospital for Women in Madras, principal of the Lady Wellington Medical School for Women, Madras, and principal of the Lady Harding Medical College in New Delhi and finally of the Christian Medical College, Vellore, South India. She inspired great confidence among her patients and many stories are told of her. On one occasion, when a village woman had hesitated at having an operation because the stars were not favourable, Hilda Lazarus replied: 'I, too, believe in stars. I work under the greatest of them all, the Star of Bethlehem. So have no fear. I shall operate tomorrow morning.'

MODERN DEVELOPMENTS

Since the time of the 1858 Medical Act medical education has changed almost out of recognition. Then the work of a body such as the Royal Society of Medicine could be conducted in only four or five specialist subsections; today it needs 34. The gradual transformation which took place in all aspects of medical training made new demands on the Christian and other philanthropists of the time, who were already carrying heavy funding schemes for the many new general and specialist hospitals. In days before government subsidies became available, further voluntary support – above what the students paid for their courses – was needed for most of the medical schools and research projects. It is amazing to observe the full extent of what the public achieved before the two world wars and the altered national circumstances made the National Health Service both inevitable and, in one sense, an ultimate fulfilment.

A major change has been the addition of a series of new medical faculties to the channels through which medical training could be gained. At the beginning of the 19th century the only universities in which medical studies could be pursued in the British Isles were in Oxford, Cambridge, the Scottish Universities, Dublin and certain private arrangements at a few London hospitals and anatomy schools. In 1826 London University was founded by the opening of University College, soon to be matched by King's College. They were both to develop medical faculties and after some years University College Hospital and King's College Hospital became available to these colleges for clinical studies. Eventually, London came to have twelve teaching hospitals. By the middle of the century, with the help in some cases of the London University system of external degrees, Medicine could be studied in Manchester, Birmingham, Sheffield, Leeds, Newcastle-on-Tyne, Bristol and Liverpool. After World War II these were joined by Nottingham, Southampton and Leicester. While instruction in the basic sciences, anatomy and physiology, was poorly paid, most of the clinical teaching in the hospitals and colleges was honorary. It is now incredible to think of the vast amount of teaching which has been voluntarily given in the medical faculties and hospitals. No doubt there was also a good deal of enlightened self-interest on the part of the consultants whose teaching impressed successive generations of general practitioners, who would in future be sending cases to them. But the evidence of biography suggests that there was also much true love of teaching and a genuine concern for the future of those in training. Also in each period there have been teachers who have specially sought to encourage the moral and spiritual health of their students. From time to time there have also been Christian movements among the medical students, for example, in organizing support for overseas medical missions.

In the late 19th and early 20th centuries, with Glasgow and Aberdeen not far behind, Edinburgh University became the centre of much energetic Christian activity among the students. There were strong student Christian Unions, especially the Student Volunteer Missionary Union, in each of the Scottish universities. In Edinburgh itself, during what came to be known as 'the year of grace 1884', many of the students were given a new practical interest in missions and eventually themselves went overseas in Christian service. The movement was strongly supported by several of the leading professors, such as A. R. Simpson, professor of gynaecology and nephew of Sir James Y. Simpson. Henry Drummond (professor of Natural Science) became the main speaker and leader. Of students in the different faculties the medicals seem to have been the most enthusiastic. Rutter Williamson, their secretary, could report for his year that from a faculty of 600 medicals, nearly 400 were members of the Edinburgh University Medical Students' Christian Association (founded in 1865).

Frederick Treves, Surgeon to the London Hospital, who on his vacations was an intrepid yachtsman, became the President of the Royal National Mission to Deepsea Fishermen. It was he who inspired one of his students, Wilfred Grenfell, to devote his life to the medical and spiritual needs of the fishermen, Eskimos and Indians on the shores of Newfoundland and Labrador. Clifford Albutt, Regius Professor of Physic at Cambridge, was constant in support of Christian activities and in encouraging Christian action by undergraduates of his acquaintance. While Thomas Barlow, physician at University College Hospital, London was specially interested in the spiritual health of his students, he also kept before the students and nurses the immense medical needs of the developing countries.

Thomas Barlow provides a good example of the part played by Christian faith in the life of a busy London physician. In a biographical sketch written for the Great Ormond Street Hospital Journal by his grandson Andrew Barlow we read: 'Religion always played an important part in Barlow's life. He had been brought up as a Wesleyan and remained faithful to that branch of the Church, but, after coming to London, Frederic Denison Maurice and William Page Roberts had much influence on his religious views and he became an admirer of the

Anglican liturgy. Like most nonconformists he felt that the sermon was a very important part of the Divine Service; in his declining years he still liked, on a Sunday, to have a sermon read to him, especially those of Jowett and Robertson. . . .' 'When I was casualty medical officer at University College Hospital, an old lady once came up for treatment. When she learned that I was related to Sir Thomas Barlow, and that he was still alive (this was in 1944) she was quite overcome with emotion, telling me that he had treated her over 50 years ago, and that he had been the leader of a Bible Class at King's Cross Chapel which she had attended. He was still remembered with devotion by members of the class and they often spoke about him. His work among the poor in the districts around University College Hospital and Great Ormond Street enabled him to gain a far greater insight into their problems than could have been achieved in the wards and outpatients department, and no doubt helped a great deal in the management and treatment of his patients.'

Between the two World Wars there were others in academic Medicine in the university cities who were similarly interested in the spiritual and moral needs of medical students. Prominent among them were Professor A. Rendle Short and Professor Duncan McCallum Blair. Rendle Short, a member of the Christian Brethren, was Professor of Surgery in the University of Bristol. Before World War I he showed his interest by organizing Sunday evening meetings for medical students in the Victoria Rooms. Later, after the war years, he worked to transfer the leadership to the students themselves and became one of the chief advocates of student-run Christian unions in the medical schools and universities. Throughout his professional life he regularly responded to invitations from their leaders to take the chair or speak at student meetings, to conduct discussions and to advise individuals. Deeply and widely read in matters concerning the Christian faith, he became one of its skilled and vigorous protagonists. As a promoter of practical action in world Medicine, he was responsible for encouraging many doctors and nurses to offer for medical missionary service. He also did much from his own financial resources to help to ensure that the missionary doctor volunteers were given adequate equipment for their tasks.

In this respect of support for medical missionaries Scotland has a proud record and a long roll of honour. The sons of the Manse and those from other Christian homes have planted across many lands pioneer Christian hospitals. Many members of the University and hospital staffs were also concerned for the future of those who would be serving at home. Duncan Blair, Regius Professor of Anatomy in the University of Glasgow and a prominent layman in the Free Church of Scotland, became intimately involved in the spiritual and moral training of medical students, both in his earlier years at King's College, London, and later when he had returned to Glasgow. His open and impressive personality attracted respect and affection from the student body. His own interest in his students was infectious and communicated itself to a number of the lecturers and professors in anatomy whom he trained. Speaking at his funeral, Sir Hector Hetherington, the Principal of the University said: 'In every university and in every generation there arise one or two men to whom it is given by some especial energy and grace to kindle and quicken the life around them. Of this good company was Duncan Blair. . . . He was devoted to the Church of his fathers. For his whole life was rooted and grounded in his religion. . . . I have not known a man happier in home, in work, in public duty or more constant in his reliance on that Christian faith which was to him the source of his serenity and strength.'

Contemporary with Duncan Blair was John Kirk, Professor of Anatomy at the Middlesex Hospital, London. A member of the Presbyterian Church of England, he had first served as one of its medical missionaries in Canton. He was a superb teacher of anatomy, especially for post-graduate students working for higher qualifications. Because of his sympathetic and sterling character and his readiness frankly to discuss any problem, he was known among his students as 'honest John'. One Christmas season a notice was fixed to the door of the Professor's room, which read: 'The Cave of Adullam. "Everyone that was in distress, and everyone that was in debt, and everyone that was discontented, gathered themselves unto him and he became a captain over them all" (1 Samuel 22:2).'

A medical specialty in which a number of Christians have become prominent is paediatrics. Among these was George Frederic Still, who gave the first description of 'Still's disease'. He was paediatric physician at King's College Hospital and Great Ormond Street Hospital, finally becoming the first Professor of Children's Diseases in London. In collaboration with Sir James Goodhart he wrote one of the earliest text-books on *The Diseases of Children* and one of the earliest histories of his specialty. A member of the Lutheran Church, he was a life-long generous supporter of many charities, and gave much of his time to his duties as honorary physician to Dr. Barnardo's Homes. Throughout his professional life, he regularly kept an appointment on Sunday afternoons. Few residents in Queen Anne Street, seeing the small figure of Sir Frederic in top hat and morning coat leaving his house, could have guessed where he was going. It was to Speaker's Corner at Marble Arch to support the Christian Evidence Society and, sometimes, to take his place on the rostrum regardless of the hecklers!

Another department which has attracted the industry of a number of Christians has been the editing of medical textbooks, several of which became best sellers. In the first half of the century two of the best known were Rose and Carless's *Manual of Surgery* (1898) and Frederick Price's *Textbook of Medicine* (1922). Professor Albert Carless of King's College Hospital saw twelve editions of his book through the press up to 1927 and further editions were supervised by Cecil P. G. Wakeley (another strong supporter of Christian and charitable causes).   Throughout his professional life, and even more after retirement, Albert Carless was identified with a variety of Christian activities and was much sought as a speaker by Christian students. It is relevant also that both Carless and Wakeley were outspokenly critical of atheistic theories of evolution, which postulate *chance* variations over very long periods of time. Carless, in addresses to students such as those on *Miracles* and *Lessons from the Human Body,* would pose the problem of a concept which required thousands of years of microscopically small chance developments which could eventually produce such a remarkable and superbly functioning organ as the human eye. Succeeding Carless's textbook, another book of surgery also ran through numerous editions and became a best seller — *A Short Practice of Surgery,* edited by R. McNeill Love (originally in collaboration with the late Hamilton Bailey). First at the London Hospital and then at the Royal Northern Hospital, 'Bobby' Love became an outstanding teacher of surgery. In his own quiet way he brought his firm Christian faith and character to bear in student and postgraduate circles.

During much the same time, Price's *Textbook of Medicine* (1922), was a best seller and went through many editions. Frederick W. Price has another claim to respect. It was Price, when cardiac physician at the Royal Northern and Heart Hospitals, who encouraged James Mackenzie when he came from Burnley to London as an unknown general practitioner hoping to interest the physicians in his work on heart disease. The London establishment was scandalized that a mere general practitioner should presume to teach it and snubbed him. It was Price who helped Mackenzie gain a footing on the staff of the Mount Vernon Hospital, Hampstead. He then let him a room at his own address at 133 Harley Street (Mackenzie 'paying for it the modest sum of £100 per annum'), and collaborated with him (also with the invaluable help of Professor Cushney, a pharmacologist) in testing the effects of several drugs on the action of the heart. Frederick Price himself became a Christian as a medical student in the Edinburgh home of Professor A. R. Simpson, nephew of Sir James Simpson of anaesthetic fame (see p. 94). Simpson for years welcomed students to a Sunday afternoon Bible Class. Between the two world wars Price, in his turn, organized a number of receptions for London medical students at his house at 133 Harley Street. After a buffet meal, before introducing the speaker, he would sometimes recall the Christian influences on the Edinburgh students of his generation and give his own short contribution.

It is perhaps here that further reference should be made to James Mackenzie, one of the outstanding band of general practitioners who have made significant contributions to medical science. From R. Macnair Wilson's life of Mackenzie *(The Beloved Physician)* we learn that it was during busy practice in Burnley that he studied the pulse and heart beat with his polygraph, before the invention of the electrocardiograph. He was assisted by Sir Arthur Keith who undertook the histological examination of the heart sections which he sent. The pathologist Wilhelm His had described the conducting bundle in the heart, but Sir Arthur had been doubtful of its existence. Stimulated, however, by papers continually sent him by Mackenzie he eventually identified it. In two of the hearts sent there had been clinically an irregularity in the auriculo-ventricular rhythm and in these he found the connecting muscle bundle largely replaced by fibrous tissue. Eventually Mackenzie's work on the heart was recognized by a post at the London Hospital. Finally he organized a cardiac research unit at St. Andrew's University.

Mackenzie's father was an elder in the United Presbyterian Church. The religious upbringing of his home, which seemed to have become somewhat dimmed in mid-life, returned fully in his closing years with a heightened love of truth, seriousness of mind, and deep sense of right and wrong. His daughter relates how she was reading to him from a life of Livingstone and he remarked, 'He was one of the happiest men in the world and I envy him with all my heart; he had complete faith'.

FUTURE SHADOWS

Medical education at the present time is confronted by a number of new problems, and not least among them is the vast amount of knowledge which has been accumulated throughout the specialties. The undergraduate medical course can now be but a brief scientific introduction to the whole field, followed by early specialization. Even more of a challenge is modern dependence at all levels, for diagnosis and treatment, on scientific mechanical aids and automation. Will the machine largely replace the physician? Will the patient become impersonal and simply a number? It is here that Christianity may be able once again to serve the sick multitudes. As in the past, it puts its pervasive emphasis on the patient as a person. Before God each individual not only has value as a person, but ideally has equal right to interest and service in time of need. It is along these lines in the Christian Churches across the world, and in appropriate new organizations, that new thought is being given to the preservation of the individuality of the patient. One of the most fruitful of these movements is that of Dr. Paul Tournier of Geneva, who organizes summer conferences on *La Médecine de la Personne*.

CHAPTER 10

MEDICAL ETHICS

IT has been a common misconception that all medical graduates in Great Britain and Ireland have subscribed to the Oath of Hippocrates. In fact, while it has been (and is) frequently referred to in lectures or commented on by medical teachers — for example in reference to the duty of confidentiality — subscription to this oath has only been required on graduation at the Scottish Universities and two others. Undoubtedly, however, this Oath, which is believed to represent the ideals of a guild of Pythagorean doctors in ancient Greece, has exercised the widest influence of any such document in the medical faculties of Europe and America.

Early in the Christian era the Church authorities questioned in the wording of the Oath the opening invocation to the heathen gods — 'I swear by Apollo physician, Asclepius, Hygeia, Panacea, and all the gods and goddesses'. They were also uneasy about several heathen practices met at certain points in Greek medical training and treatment. In the early Middle Ages alternative Christian wordings appeared at the beginning of the Oath, for example 'Blessed be God the Father of our Lord Jesus Christ, I lie not . . .'. It is in this form that the Oath is used for a graduation ceremony in Scotland. During most of the Christian era the ethics of the doctor-patient relationship have rested on general Christian ethics based on the Ten Commandments of the Old Testament and the Golden Rule of the New Testament — 'in everything do to others what you would have them do to you' (Matthew 7:12).

Depending on the changes in the prevailing cultural, religious and social conditions, there have been roughly four main periods in the history of medical ethics — (1) *Ancient,* up to AD 500; (ii) *Medieval,* AD 500-1500; (iii) *Modern,* AD 1500-1800 (to the French Revolution); and (iv) *Contemporary.* In the first period there was in Christian circles an uneasy compromise between the Graeco-Roman and the Christian traditions, with the Church gradually gaining the ascendancy. In the second period Medicine in Christian regions came gradually under the care of the monasteries, the priest-physicians and the universities, and all of these were dominated by the Church. In the third, the forces of the Renaissance and Reformation in the Protestant countries greatly reduced the medieval Church's dominance and brought medical practice largely into the hands of laymen. While Christian ethics still exercised a powerful influence, there were other contenders for the guidance of professional etiquette and ethics. Finally, today, Christian ethics has to meet scientific humanism as its most powerful rival in determining the ethical issues confronting the profession.

THE CHRISTIAN TRADITION

Throughout the Christian era there have been prominent Christian practitioners who have thought and written on the problems of professional conduct, for example Ambroĩse Paré and Thomas Browne of Norwich, the latter in his *Confessio Medici* (1643) and *Christian Morals* (posthumous 1716). Similarly, the Puritan physician Thomas Sydenham, the English Hippocrates, in the course of his clinical writings emphasizes the accountability of a medical practitioner 'to the Supreme Judge' and the need for a physician to show compassion for his fellow mortals when he reflects that he himself is also mortal. More systematic presentations of the problems were put forward by John Gregory, Professor of Physic in Edinburgh, in *Duties and Qualifications of a Physician* (1772) and by Thomas Percival in his *Medical Ethics* (1803).

Percival, a physician of the Manchester Royal Infirmary, was a staunch Dissenter and product of the famous Puritan dissenting academy at Warrington.   Excluded by his nonconformity from Oxford and Cambridge, he qualified medically at Edinburgh.   Returning to Manchester he is soon found prominent among the active philanthropists who were endeavouring to mitigate the worst effects of the increasing industrialization, to bring relief to the poor, and to instal better sanitation. He proved to be a man of great integrity, charming manner and with exemplary relations with his medical colleagues. It was, therefore, natural that he should be asked at a time of crisis and dispute on the staff of the Infirmary to draw up 'a scheme of professional conduct relative to the hospitals and other charities'. While the result, perhaps inevitably, was more concerned with etiquette between doctors (than with ethics proper), it represented the first effective step towards a more satisfactory modern professional 'code'. Percival's 'Code' had great influence in the U.S.A. where it was unrivalled until the American Medical Association and State Associations began to compile their own.

Throughout the increasingly rapid changes of the late 19th and 20th centuries, the contributions to a reconsideration of medical ethics came mainly from individuals. There was, however, a general rise of standards in all aspects of medical practice and the pervasive influence of the Christian faith must be given much of the credit. The position is well illustrated by the evidence of the effects of their Christian education on the outlook of a distinguished American physician and in the life of a Scottish general practitioner.

One of the chief exemplars of the high ethical standards prevailing in the early part of the 20th century was Richard C. Cabot of Boston, Massachusetts. He was honorary consulting physician at the Massachusetts General Hospital and Professor of Clinical Medicine at the Harvard Medical School. He was well respected for his skill in the art of diagnosis. He was the originator of what became popularly known as 'clinico-pathological conferences', in which case histories were frankly compared with subsequent pathological or postmortem findings. His book on *Differential Diagnosis* went into ten editions.

His sturdily independent character began to give its attention to some of the more stubborn problems of social ethics. He was responsible for the introduction of a new service by trained hospital personnel who are today known as medical social workers. Among his 23 books and many journal articles are several works on ethics which have had a wide circulation. Best known of these are: *What Men Live By* (1911), *The Meaning of Right and Wrong* (1933), *The Art of Ministering to the Sick* (1936) and *Honesty* (1938).

In the last of these Cabot makes his outlook clear from the outset. 'For at least half a century I have found honesty a most interesting subject. Next to food and shelter it seems to be one of our greatest needs. Without some of it we cannot live together, work together, or play together successfully. Deceit disorganizes and discourages human endeavour. Moreover, we show at times a deep hunger for sincerity and reality in our fellow men. We want a genuineness in them that parallels the genuineness of nature. . . . Yet we do not behave as if *between men* we valued honesty supremely. In Medicine and social work I have been amazed at the degree of acquiescence in dishonesty. We think we can make exceptions to the rule of truthfulness though nature makes none. Yet we are not sure of this, for we are forever eager to discuss the question: "Is it ever right to lie?" ' Richard Cabot's emphasis on truthfulness and his call for rock-like professional integrity brought a healthy challenge to the English-speaking professional world.

ETHICS IN GENERAL PRACTICE

Since the chief medical advances and crucial steps in medical care have taken place in the hospitals, we need to be reminded that all over the world much of the best Medicine is offered daily by thousands of competent and hard working general practitioners. In matters of day-to-day ethics much depends on their commonsense and reliability. A number of attractive biographies have given some glimpses of the challenges, hardships and rewards of the older-type practitioner.

A good example is found in *Leaves from the Life of a Country Doctor,* edited by Rutherford Crockett. It highlights the work of Clement Bryce Gunn of Peebles, a boyhood friend of John Buchan (Lord Tweedsmuir). Its pages are studded with descriptions of midnight journeys through flood and tempest to distant farms and lonely crofts. The driving force behind Dr Gunn's dedication is given in his own words.

'*March 1893.* An inestimable benefit to our sick poor has just been inaugurated here in the establishment of a Queen's nurse. We doctors are greatly indebted to these nurses for much valuable help and observation, and the poor have a greatly improved chance of recovery owing to their skilful, efficient and devoted nursing. It is borne in upon me that unless one is animated by the spirit of Christ one cannot be successful either as a doctor or as a nurse. One must have spiritual insight if one is to approach the poor, the sick, the destitute and the fallen. Upheld by this inner vision, one can find courage, inspiration, and determination to fight disease; not otherwise.'

'*Hogmanay 1894.* At four in the morning I was called to attend a maternity case, which I am aware will develop into a bad debt, though the patient's husband is in work, and could pay if willing. My bad debts during the past year or two have amounted to 40%. Nevertheless, some time ago, I resolved that I would attend all poor patients who applied, and refuse none. My reason is this: I earnestly endeavour, so far as I can, to approach the suffering poor in the spirit of Christ. I have no money to give them; nor am I fitted to offer them the consolation of good words spoken in season. But this one thing I can and will do: attend the poor without payment; and that must be my religious duty henceforward. On this the last night of the year, I reaffirm the above decision in the spirit of earnest resolve.'

THE CRISIS OF THE MID-TWENTIETH CENTURY

Up until 1914 the spiritual and moral outlook in the medical professions of the West were comparatively homogeneous. Though many of the doctors were not practising Christians, the influence of the Churches and the uniting effect of Christian education gave general similarity of outlook in these matters. Many non-Christians unconsciously followed the prevailing general principles of Christian ethics. But two devastating world wars, a great acceleration in the process of secularization and the steady growth in education circles of articulate scientific humanism rapidly brought about a very different situation. Perhaps even more disturbing for medical ethics was the growth in ability of the more progressive members of the profession to perform various procedures in relation to the human body which had never before been within the bounds of possibility. In a comparatively few years the whole profession was confronted by the crucial question: 'Is what is now feasible necessarily and ethically right?'

During recent years such a question has made its way into almost every department of medical ethics, affecting procedures from the beginning to the end of human life. Bioengineering has developed yet further startling possibilities. Geneticists, surgeons and others have been more than ready to play God. So the profession, and the nation as a whole, must now come to terms with the stark necessity of adjusting the relationship between feasibility and rectitude in the conduct of medical practice. Codes such as that of Hippocrates have been long out of date and the controlling bodies of the world's medical professions have had to give urgent reconsideration to almost every aspect of medical ethics.

The agreed statements which have gained most widespread international support are those of the World Medical Association as set out in its International Code of Medical Ethics and the Declaration of Geneva (1948). This has been supplemented at each subsequent international meeting of the Association by additional agreed statements on further problems — at Helsinki (1964) on Clinical Research, Sydney (1968) on Death, Oslo (1970) on Therapeutic Abortion, Tokyo (1975) on Torture and Hawaii (1977) on Psychiatry. There is little doubt that in the thinking and discussions of these assemblies the Christian outlook has been well represented.

It is at such points in the developing traditions of the world's medical professions that the influence of Christians has been strong and has proved its value. Over against an agnostic or atheistic scientific humanism the Christian faith presents a world and life view of personal Theism. It lays down such principles as man's accountability to God, his responsibility to search for and to speak the truth, his obligation to respect life and his duty to do for his neighbour what he would like done for himself. These ideals are very difficult of realization and they can only be approached when Christian faith is strong. In the next few years it will be seen how far they can be preserved and achieved.

The comprehensive and far-reaching nature of such ideals in the present confused situation in medical ethics can best be illustrated by a reproduction of one of the Christian statements. The following is a Christian Affirmation adopted for its members by the (British) Christian Medical Fellowship:

CHRISTIAN ETHICS IN MEDICAL PRACTICE

A Christian doctor gratefully accepts the heritage of knowledge passed down from the earliest times by the great pioneers and teachers of Medicine. Medical practice, however, requires more than knowledge and technical skills. In personal relations and in attitude to work he will make it his aim to be guided by the teaching of Jesus Christ as recorded in the Bible. Central to this is the unequivocal declaration — 'The Lord your God is the only Lord; love the Lord your God with all your heart, and with all your soul, and with all your mind, and with all your strength . . . and love your neighbour as yourself (Mark 12:30, 31).

The following are some of the applications of this principle:

A Christian Affirmation

I acknowledge that in all I do I am accountable to God. I shall endeavour, therefore, to conduct my professional life in accordance with the standards of Christ.

In relation to Human Life

To acknowledge that God is the Creator and the Lord of all life.

To recognize that man is unique, being made 'in the image of God', and that he cannot be healthy in body and mind unless he lives in harmony with the natural world around him, neither ignoring nor exploiting it.

To maintain the deepest respect for individual human life from its beginning to its close, including the helpless, handicapped or advanced in age.

To use only those drugs and procedures which are for the benefit of the patient, avoiding all that may harm him.

To promote a sense of vocation in the work by which men live and serve one another, and to honour and recommend the Creator's rule of one day's rest in seven.

To uphold marriage as a lasting bond, being the divinely appointed means for the care of children, the security of the family and the stability of society.

To regard sexual intercourse as admissible only within the marriage relationship; and, hence, to advocate premarital continence and marital fidelity.

In relation to Professional Work

To give effective service to those seeking medical care irrespective of age, race, creed, politics, social status or the circumstances which may have contributed to their illness.

To serve the patient according to his need, declining to be influenced by motives of self-interest or gain.

To respect his privacy, opinions and personal feelings and to keep his confidence.

To speak truthfully to him, bearing in mind my own fallibility.

To work constructively with my colleagues, as opportunity and ability permit, in the advance of medical science throughout the world.

To recognize, when the interests of the community conflict with those of the individual, that the doctor's first duty is to his patient.

To deal honestly with my professional and administrative colleagues, and to fulfil the just requirements of the State.

CHAPTER 11

THE DEVELOPMENT OF MODERN NURSING

THROUGHOUT history the Christian church has made its main impact in two ways. Firstly when the church itself, or a section of it, has set up institutions to forward its ideals, and secondly when private individual Christians working in the secular sphere have brought to their work the inspiration and insights which they had learned in the church. Second in importance only to the great technical and scientific advances in Medicine of the 19th century was the foundation of nursing as a profession. Without it the great advances in surgery, and all the careful observation and care of patients required by modern therapeutics, would have been impossible. As in the 18th century Christian men played a large part in founding hospitals throughout the land, so in the 19th the provision of nurses for those hospitals was largely the gift of the Christian Church.

However, each century does not always continue the advances made in the past and the work of the medieval sisterhoods and of Vincent de Paul had largely been forgotten. So much so that Dickens could caricature at least some of the midwives and nurses of his age in the figures of Sairey Gamp and Betsy Trotwood. A brief reference to the earlier forms of nursing will provide a necessary perspective.

THE DARK AND MEDIEVAL AGES

In the late Roman Empire, when the decrees of Constantine had permitted greater liberty of action to Christians, the Church is found organizing its deaconesses, widows and unmarried women into teams for elementary nursing and social service. Some of the richer Roman matrons — and later even queens — are found leading the way. Then, when monastic institutions had grown in number and some of the monks, such as the Benedictines, had become engaged in medical services, some of the women's convents are found similarly employed. Little in detail is known of what this meant and some of it would seem to have been more in the nature of social service than nursing; but the few extant records indicate due appreciation by the people of the proto-hospitals and the home visits.

At the time of the medieval military nursing orders, such as the Knights Hospitallers of St. John of Jerusalem (Rhodes and Malta), the Teutonic Knights (Deutsche Orden) and the Knights of St. Lazarus (for leprosy cases), there were corresponding orders for women nurses under the title 'Sisters'. In these cases — or some of them — the women seem to have had their own women's hospitals. Later in the Middle Ages, there were a number of women's nursing orders such as the Franciscan Tertianes, the Poor Clares, the Sisterhood of the Common Life and the Oblates of Florence. Perhaps historically the most interesting, however, are the Sisters of the Hôtel Dieu in Paris, who appear first as a group of volunteers put in charge of the sick at the Hôtel Dieu in AD 650. Their tradition has survived into the present. They are believed to be the oldest of any order of nuns who are devoted solely to nursing.

The nearest approach to more modern methods of nursing came from the remarkably far-sighted work of a simple parish priest in the 17th century, St Vincent de Paul, in Paris. Distressed beyond measure by what he saw in the poor quarters of Paris, he planned and put into operation a movement for hospital reform, social service, education, manual training and every possible inducement to self-help, which were years ahead of his time. For the nursing needs of the people, with the help of some of the Sisters from the Hôtel Dieu, he organized devout laywomen, together with girls from country parishes, into a nursing order primarily for home visiting, under the name Dames de Charité.

The Dames were based on the Hôtel Dieu and gradually on other hospitals of Paris so that their more serious cases could be brought into the hospital wards. It is interesting, too — in view of what is still found to be the optimum load for a visiting nurse — that Vincent de Paul recommended that none of the Sisters should accept responsibility for more than eight nursing cases. The Sisters of Charity spread to other countries, became the best loved of the orders, and have come down to the present time. It is also salutary to note that, whereas the provision for the British Army in the Crimean campaign was at the outset so abysmal, the French forces were accompanied by a suitable unit of the Sisters of Charity.

In Roman Catholic regions most of the existing nursing orders continued uninterrupted beyond the Reformation, but in Protestant lands the dissolution of the monasteries and convents left a considerable gap in the nursing services. In no country was this so pronounced as in England. While there may have been an increase in self-help and home nursing, many of the hospitals were for a time closed. It was some years before the civic and other secular authorities began to assume more appropriate responsibility for social needs. In any real meaning of the term 'modern', as applied to nursing, the hospital had to await the 19th century.

KAISERSWERTH, GERMANY

The first step in the right direction came from Theodor Fliedner, a Lutheran pastor at Kaiserswerth on the Rhine. He revived the ancient term 'deaconess' (from the Greek *diakonis,* a servant or minister) and applied it to his circle of Protestant women who wished to dedicate themselves to the care of the sick and education of neglected children. He himself, on visiting England, had been inspired by Elizabeth Fry's work in women's prisons. Fliedner and his wife first opened a small refuge for discharged prisoners. Then in 1836, having seen the work of evangelical deaconesses in Holland, they opened a small hospital for the poor.

The nursing was undertaken by young women. The first group were six in number and they divided the work between them, changing duty periods regularly in order to gain wider experience. Frederike Fliedner taught them practical nursing and her husband taught Christian doctrine and ethics. Nurses took the state examination in pharmacy. They were soon nursing in the city hospital of Elberfeld. Their work grew and Kaiserswerth soon found itself the motherhouse for many daughter-houses in Germany and the countries adjoining. In due time Elizabeth Fry and Florence Nightingale visited Kaiserswerth and for some three months the latter took part in the training.

THE BRITISH ISLES

In England Elizabeth Fry (née Gurney) continued John Howard's work among prisoners. She was a Quaker and cared not only for the physical welfare of those she visited in prison, but read the Bible to the female prisoners in Newgate Street gaol. Her husband was a 'minister' among the Quakers and a noted speaker. Following the example of Pastor Fliedner, she formed an association of ladies who became known as the 'Fry nurses'. They visited the sick poor in their homes. Although they had comparatively little nursing training, they each were sent to Guy's Hospital daily for a few months to learn the elements of their work.

In Catholic Ireland Mary Aikenhead formed the Irish Sisters of Charity and Catherine McAuley the Sisters of Mercy. Members of both these organizations nursed the cholera patients during the outbreak in Dublin. This was a courageous act for by then the highly contagious nature of cholera was known. Some of the sisters from Ireland also joined Florence Nightingale in the Crimea. Additional nursing orders began to appear. For example, within the Anglican community, the Rev. E. B. Pusey prompted the formation of a guild of Anglican Sisters of Mercy. These, however, had no hospital training and their work was primarily to visit the sick in their homes. John Neale (known today as the writer of such hymns as 'O happy band of pilgrims' and 'Art thou weary') founded in 1855 the Anglican Sisterhood of St. Margaret which was concerned in both the education of girls and the care of the sick. They did loyal service in a smallpox epidemic at Haggerston in 1866. These two orders might be regarded as the forerunners of the district nursing service, for their domiciliary visits were very similar in nature.

Hospital nursing became the sphere of activity for St. John's House and to a lesser degree of the All Saints Sisterhood. St. John's House, founded in 1848, was the first purely nursing order in the Church of England. It was an important landmark in English nursing history. At first their nurses were trained either at the Middlesex or the Westminster Hospitals, but from 1855 they were also trained at King's College Hospital which at that time was situated just behind the site of the Royal College of Surgeons of England in Lincoln's Inn Fields. From 1856 they undertook the whole of the nursing at King's College Hospital, while the All Saints Sisterhood, founded in 1851, took over all the nursing at University College Hospital. The use of the word 'sister' to denote those in charge of the nursing in a ward is a relic of the day when ward nursing was done by such Christian nursing orders.

THE FIRST NURSING MOVEMENT

Florence Nightingale appeared against such a background. Lytton Strachey in his *Great Victorians* has not been over-complimentary of her, but although in real life she may not quite have matched the popular image of 'the lady of the lamp', a difficult personality such as hers was needed to bring about the reforms which she managed to achieve. Born in Florence (hence her name), she took a passionate interest in nursing at a time when it was not quite an occupation for 'ladies'. After a short spell in Germany at Kaiserswerth, she returned to England in 1851 and was appointed head of a nursing home for invalid gentlewomen. In 1854, with the outbreak of the Crimean War, her opportunity arrived. As reports were received of the dreadful conditions which accentuated the plight of the wounded in that campaign, public opinion in England was roused and she was despatched to the Crimea with her band of nurses. They descended on Scutari. She not only organized the nursing there but dealt with problems of hygiene and the ordering of supplies. Typically, among her early orders was one for 300 scrubbing brushes. There being no night nurses in the wards, she herself nightly toured the four miles of beds, lamp in hand, to comfort the sick and wounded. Finally, so that the scientific side should not be neglected, she took a house at her own expense to serve as a laboratory and a dissecting room. This small sideline was destined to become the nucleus of the medical school of the Royal Army Medical Corps.

Florence Nightingale made an enormous impact both in the field and at home. In 1856, with the war ended, she returned to England to continue her battle for better nursing. She had what was in those days called a 'neurasthenia' and retired, hermit-like, to her room where, most unhermit-like, she continued the fight. We can only conjecture what diagnosis a modern psychiatrist would have suggested. She interviewed, she wrote letters, she advised those in authority, and she exercised to the full the power her fame had brought her. Finally her dream of a nursing school materialized, with Miss Wardroper at St. Thomas's Hospital proving to be a loyal and cooperative ally in the beginnings of what became the Nightingale Nurses Home.

Her achievements were outstanding, her limitations (dare we say failings?) were all too obvious, but that she had experienced a 'call' to some higher task she herself affirmed: 'God called me to His service Feb. 7 1837'. Her stay at Kaiserswerth with its deep Christian background was a turning point in her life. Afterwards she referred to it as her 'spiritual home' although she was not uncritical of the hospital side of the Kaiserswerth enterprise. One church leader described her as belonging to 'a sect which is unfortunately a very rare one — the sect of the Good Samaritan'. Difficult as she was, 'she was a devoutly religious woman and always regarded nursing as a vocation and not as a trade'. She grasped the New Testament ideal of caring for the sick and interpreted it in secular terms, showing that it was not only deaconesses who were capable of making good nurses. Coming from a well-to-do family she had the added motive that the rich and privileged should serve the poor and needy. 'Inasmuch as ye did it unto the least of these my brethren, ye did it unto me.'

OTHER EXPRESSIONS OF THE MOVEMENT

Ellen Ranyard, in the first instance, founded a mission in order to distribute Bibles to the poor and by 1879 she had some 170 Bible women working with her. She then came to see the medical needs of the underprivileged and arranged for her workers to be trained as nurses. By 1868 she had started such nursing training and soon had 80 of her women attending the sick poor. The Ranyard Nurses remained active even after her death and until the beginning of World War II.

The German Hospital was founded to meet the needs of Germans living in London, many of whom did not have a competent grasp of the English language. A German pastor and the physician Dr. J. H. C. Freund combined to make an appeal to their homeland for the finance and in 1845 it was ready to receive patients. Having only 36 beds at first, it limited its intake to German-speaking patients. It also had an outpatient department and the whole institution was run on the lines of a British voluntary hospital. Originally nurses were enlisted from Pastor Fliedner's Deaconess Schools and this may explain why its standards of cleanliness and its mortality rates in the pre-Nightingale era compared very favourably with other British hospitals. By the time of the outbreak of World War II the hospital had expanded to 224 beds. In due course it was assimilated into the National Health Service, leaving only its name as a reminder of its origin.

Across the Continent the work of the Kaiserswerth deaconesses spread and many other women members of the Protestant Churches were trained both for spiritual work in association with the Christian ministry and also for nursing and social services. The developments at Kaiserswerth were eagerly studied and some of the senior deaconesses were sent to assist in the setting up of similar training centres in the countries of central and northern Europe. Soon the Lutherans and Anglicans were joined by the Presbyterian, Methodist and other Christian Churches in accepting the concept of nursing sisters and taking action each in their distinctive ways.

Nowhere was interest more enthusiastic and the ultimate impact more extensive than in North America. In French Canada there had already been a considerable amount of work done by French nuns who had been sent from France, and the same was true of the Roman Catholic areas of the United States. Eventually there were to be impressive Hôtels Dieu in Quebec and Montreal and in some of the U.S. cities, such as the Charity Hospital of New Orleans. At an early date the Quakers and Presbyterians in Philadelphia were greatly concerned about public health, nursing and social conditions. The Philadelphia General Hospital (known as Blockley and founded as early as 1731) was eventually to become one of the chief centres of the new humanitarian influences. The religious circles of Pennsylvania and Massachusetts were two of the chief power houses in the modern nursing movement of the late 19th century.

There was another phase in the movement. It was not long before what had been, in origin and support, a religiously motivated movement was joined by a second on more secular and public lines. The fame and public activity of Florence Nightingale led in Britain to a national and then to an international interest. The project of the reform of nursing – and in some of the countries of trained nursing of any kind – became a priority. The Nightingale standards were adopted in many countries as an ideal and a pattern. Sisters trained at St. Thomas's were welcomed everywhere to lend their assistance in the various new national training schemes. Many are the reports of the outstanding work done. For example, the transformation of the old Blockley in Philadelphia, and its subsequent influence on other institutions, was directly due to St. Thomas's trained Alice Fisher, accompanied by another 'Nightingale'. For many years she was the greatly loved Matron and idol of the Blockley.

It is not without significance that the two streams – religious and secular – came together at international levels just when they did, for it was about that time that the widespread building of new general and specialist hospitals was being embarked upon. So when the demand came for large battalions of rightly motivated and more scientifically trained nurses, to a large extent they were ready. Yet whatever may be the future spiritual outlook in the history of the medical profession, nothing should be allowed to detract from the debt owed to the Christian churches for the availability of the thousands of new nurses at that time.

The welcome to the Kaiserswerth Sisters and the 'Nightingales' was not only a matter of course in the West; they were also well received in a number of countries where other religions were in control. Many were the tributes from the beneficiaries to the quality of the new nurses and the effect of their teaching and example. There is a well authenticated story of an experienced Hindu surgeon from Bombay who arrived unannounced and asked to spend the day at a prominent mission hospital to see the work. He was allowed to spend the day as he wished. When he left he said quietly to the surgeon in charge, 'Do you know what has impressed me most today? While I was watching you operating, a nurse in the distance carrying in a tray of sterilized instruments dropped one on to the floor. She was out of your sight, but came on and put the tray down and then went back, picked up the instrument, and took it back to be re-sterilized. How do you produce such integrity in your Nurses?'

THE SECOND MODERN NURSING MOVEMENT

In the closing years of the 19th century most of the energies of the nurses in Britain were directed towards improving standards in the existing institutions and ensuring that the new hospitals started at adequate levels. Due to the rapid advances in surgery and growth of the medical sciences, there was need for constant review of the subjects needing to be included in the courses of training. Hospital managements began to confer, and in 1886 a national Hospitals Association came into being to facilitate such consultations. One of its first acts was to set up a committee to explore the desirability of establishing a national register of nurses. On such a register only those applicants would be placed who had completed a recognized nursing training. On various grounds a number of nurses (and doctors) were strongly opposed to such a proposal. Those opposed included the formidable Florence Nightingale, who was afraid that a new 'professionalism' might dilute bedside nursing. She influenced the views of a number of powerful friends and as a result action was delayed for some 30 years.

However, among those working to secure professional status for nurses there was another able, farsighted and determined woman. She was also capable of a long campaign. What she achieved summarizes the main results of the second nurses' movement.

Ethel Gordon Manson was the daughter of a doctor practising in Morayshire, who died in her infancy. Her mother's second marriage to a Nottingham Member of Parliament brought her to England. After training as a nurse at the Children's Hospital, Nottingham, and then at Manchester Royal Infirmary, she became a Sister at the London Hospital. Her remarkable organizing ability was soon discovered and at the early age of 24 she found herself appointed Matron and Superintendent of Nurses at St Bartholomew's Hospital. Her direct nursing career was terminated by marriage in 1887 to a London gynaecologist. This, however, seems only to have released her for her life's work and it was as Mrs Bedford Fenwick that she became known to the nursing world.

When the Hospital Association hesitated to proceed to ask for professional status she resigned from it and founded in 1887 the British Nurses'

Association. Six years later this new body became the first women's professional organization to receive a royal charter. Mrs. Bedford Fenwick then proceeded to work for Government legislation to buttress the professional status of nurses by establishing a national register. This, after a long struggle, was finally gained by the passing of the Nurses Registration Act in 1919. Meanwhile she had brought into being a Matrons' Council of Great Britain and the National Council of Nurses of Great Britain. Finally in 1926 she had started the British College of Nurses. Meanwhile she had acquired the journal *The Nursing Record* (of which she changed the name to *British Journal of Nursing*) and she continued to edit it for many years.

The situation in most of the other Western countries followed a somewhat similar course and the organizational battles of the British nurses were of considerable interest to the nurses of other countries. It is not, therefore, surprising to find that Mrs. Bedford Fenwick reached the summit of her career by becoming the founder and President of the International Council of Nurses. This held its first world congress in Buffalo, U.S.A., in 1901. When she was a youthful matron of St. Bartholomew's, the nursing world was a series of groups of well-meaning helpers of widely different training and skills. Some were good, but others had had little training. She left nursing a well trained profession of good minimum standards and which had many members who were very good.

It is not possible here to do justice to the worldwide epic of modern nursing. It is filled with examples of the most amazing industry, personal devotion and heroic self-sacrifice. The full story could only be told in a countless succession of individual portraits. They would have to open with an example such as that of Mary Robinson who started district nursing in Liverpool. She was encouraged and supported by William Rathbone, a Unitarian merchant, to nurse the poor of an underprivileged district of the city in their own homes. She had wished to give up the attempt after one month, broken-hearted by the unbelievable misery she found. Spurred on, however, by Rathbone she stuck to it and blazed the trail. When William Rathbone applied to St Thomas's and King's College Hospital for nurses to carry the project further, the reply was that all those they had trained were in demand for leadership elsewhere and there were more requests than they could hope to meet. He then offered to build a Nurses' Home and training centre attached to the Liverpool Royal Infirmary. The nurses in Liverpool soon found that a number of the cases of serious illness needed hospital treatment and the question of stepping up standards in the Poor Law institutions became urgent. William

Rathbone offered to support a leader and twelve 'Nightingales' from St. Thomas's, who would be joined to twelve locally trained nurses.

Miss Nightingale's choice for the key position of superintendent of the Liverpool nurses fell on Agnes Jones, a beautiful Irish girl and daughter of an army colonel from Londonderry. She had trained at Kaiserswerth, Miss Ranyard's Bible Mission in East London, St Thomas's and the Great Northern Hospital in London. She took over a crowded Brownlow Hill Infirmary, full of men in all forms of mental and physical degradation sleeping two or three in a single bed. In her first letter she described it as being 'like Dante's Inferno'. She first got the Governor to introduce various forms of orderly duty and work, and within a month 200 malingerers found it convenient to take their leave. To train pauper women to help was found to be quite impractical and useless as they quickly spent their pay getting hopelessly drunk. She gradually introduced trained women to the Infirmary and succeeded against all expectations in completely transforming Poor Law nursing. Alas, in her third year Agnes Jones died from typhus fever acquired from a home visit.

The story could then go on to spectacular successes such as those of the American nursing sister, Emma D. Cushman. Trained at the Paterson General Hospital, New Jersey, she was a Christian missionary in Turkey at the outbreak of World War I. She declined to leave the country and eventually became the acting consul for 17 nations. The *American Journal of Nursing* in 1931 reported how 'This dauntless missionary nurse became father and mother to tens of thousands of the war's victims — the Kut-el-Amara British prisoners; the interned Roman Catholic priests and nuns; prisoners and refugees from all corners of the sultan's domains; and thousands of Armenian orphans and deportees. Upon the assurance of Ambassador Morgenthau before the curtain of silence enveloped Turkey that her drafts would be honoured, she wrote in simple faith cheques for over a million dollars for carrying on her unparalleled work of ministry and relief. She was nurse, almoner, administrator, priest, financier and statesman. History has no equal to Miss Cushman's work at Konia; only those whose lives she saved can understand its magnitude.' At the end of the war, during the resettlement of 22,000 Christian children in other parts of the Near East, Emma Cushman went with 3000 of them to Greece. She died in Egypt in 1930.

CHAPTER 12

WIDER ASPECTS OF MEDICAL CARE

MOST advances in medical science have come through the initiatives of those who were specially trained for it, but there have been a number of beneficent discoveries which originated with those who were, from the medical point of view, laymen. Several examples have already been given in earlier chapters, such as the fascination with optics shown in the Middle Ages by Bishop Robert Grosseteste and his disciple Roger Bacon. Again, it was Louis Pasteur — a Catholic biochemist — who established the basis for Lister's antiseptic surgery, while it was the work of two chemists, Sir Humphry Davy a Methodist, and Michael Faraday from a Lowlands Presbyterian sect, who opened the way for anaesthetics.

THE CONTRIBUTIONS OF LAYMEN

Medicine certainly does not exist in a vacuum. It draws on the work of the basic sciences and sometimes also contributes its findings to them. Three examples are given below of laymen who have helped to lay the foundation of some of the branches of Medicine.

Gregor Mendel, the son of a peasant farmer, entered the Augustinian order at Brunn in Silesia and was ordained to the priesthood in 1847. His scientific abilities were recognized and he was given leave to study science at Vienna from 1851-1853. Returning to his monastery he was made abbot. Among other activities he quietly studied the propagation of sweet peas in the monastery garden. His success depended on the fact that he concentrated attention on single characteristics of the plants which he kept under observation. From these he ventured to enunciate laws which govern the transmission of given traits from generation to generation, formulating a theory of dominance. He published his findings in 1865 in an obscure journal, *The Proceedings of the Brno Natural History Society,* where they remained unnoticed until, in 1900, the paper was discovered independently by three botanists. Later the modern concept of the gene was introduced to explain his work and from this both the sciences of genetics and the discipline of genetic counselling have grown.

The founder of the Red Cross, Henri Dunant, was not a doctor but a Genevan business man and philanthropist. A member of the Reformed Church, he was a very active Christian. In 1859 he happened to be travelling past the area where the battle of Solferino had just been fought. He was appalled by the sight of the aftermath on the battlefield and set to work to assist the wounded and dying. In 1862 he published a book *A Memory of Solferino* in which he not only related his experiences, but suggested the formation of voluntary aid societies to assist the army medical services. He also proposed an international convention for the protection of the wounded, the buildings that housed them and the staff who attended them. In 1863 he was one of a committee of five which took the steps which led to the formation of the International Red Cross Society. In 1901 he was the first recipient of the Nobel Prize for Peace.

In the history of institutions and movements it is easy to overlook the importance of adequate finance and the support which wealthy men have given to make possible some of the modern discoveries. Hence the importance of John Davison Rockefeller. He was a noted business man who made vast sums of money through the Standard Oil Company which he, together with his brother William, founded. For a while this company exercised a virtual monopoly of the oil supplies to North America. He revealed himself as a generous philanthropist and eventually gave away over 500 million dollars. Among similar charities he founded the Rockefeller Foundation in 1913 to 'promote the well being of mankind' and through it he gave large sums to medical research and medical foundations. He came to exercise a marked influence on the growth of 20th century Medicine. Rockefeller was a Baptist and some of his donations were also given to religious causes, for example to medical missions.

It is of interest to recall the achievements of Christian doctors in spheres other than that of Medicine — a salutary reminder to us all that we must be interested in the milieu in which our patients live out their lives, as well as in their complaints. Son of a rice farmer, Sun Yat Sen was sent to school in Honolulu run by an Anglican bishop. Later, in Hong Kong, he became the first graduate in the school of medicine run by Dr. (later Sir) James Cantlie. He travelled widely and was kidnapped by the Chinese legation in London while walking down Devonshire Street on his way to church. After his release he became the Provisional President of the Republic of China. In 1912, after a varied story of exile and return, he again attempted to unify his country, but unfortunately he died of cancer of the stomach. Thus it was a Christian medical man who became one of the early pioneers among those who attempted to bring China out of the medieval age.

THE EVANGELICALS AND SOCIAL NEEDS

Nineteenth century Britain saw a nationwide movement which succeeded in mobilizing the Christians to confront the appalling social needs which had followed in the wake of the Industrial Revolution. Most of the Churches were involved, but it was the Evangelicals in the Church of England and the Methodists who were most often found in the vanguard. A stimulating and discerning account of some of the reforming organizations has been given in Kathleen Heasman's *Evangelicals in Action*.

The strength and extent of the movement was astonishing. It seems as if at that time a voluntary society was started to meet almost every conceivable need. But the main force of the movement was directed towards offering elementary education and meeting the chief social evils, such as drunkenness. Perhaps part of the movement's main value was the light which it threw into all the dark corners, revealing the full extent of the national task. The amount which it raised in voluntary subscriptions was formidable and the full total of volunteers who offered for the many arduous tasks quite incredible.

In summarizing the nature and spheres of influence of the long list of evangelical societies Dr Heasman writes: 'A very large number were Christian missions for the general benefit of the poor. Many were for children, and for the first time the needs of the teenager began to be considered. Attention was paid to the misfits in society, the drunkard, the criminal, and the prostitute, usually with the purpose of helping them to conform, and it was gradually realized that aftercare was as crucial a part of the social work as the giving of immediate help. Finally, among the organizations for the benefits of small groups of people with some particular need, the Evangelicals tended to concentrate upon the soldier and sailor, the railwayman and the navvy, the needlewoman and the business girl, and the domestic servant.'

For our present purposes, where medical needs are the centre of interest, reference will be made to the medical missions, the medical work of the Salvation Army, the homes for orphans, the efforts to reduce drunkenness and to give help to the handicapped.

MEDICAL MISSIONS IN THE INNER CITIES

While the Victorian Church contributed large sums towards the support of mission hospitals overseas, it did not neglect the poor on its doorstep. Among the crowds in the central areas of the industrial towns were many who could afford neither to see a doctor nor to pay for any drugs which might be prescribed. Few doctors were attracted to practise — or could have survived — in such areas. The conditions, however, stirred the Christian medical conscience and in many of the underprivileged areas medical missions were established so that, at least, needs at the family doctor level could be met. As circumstances changed many of these missions became extinct but a few remained to continue under the National Health Service with something of their original aim and motivation.

The first such oasis to open its doors in the London area was the London Medical Mission, a non-denominational mission situated in Endell Street just off Drury Lane. It was set up in 1871 by Dr. George Saunders who had been deeply impressed on hearing of the city medical missions in Edinburgh, Liverpool and Manchester. In one of the early circulars written to gain support is written: 'The miserable condition of the poor, morally, physically and spiritually, is a loud call to all Christians for hearty cooperation in the promotion of a work so peculiarly fitted to meet the urgent requirements of the dark places of our great cities.' After a time a holiday home was opened at Folkestone to which convalescent cases could be sent. Towards the close of the century a branch was opened in Lambeth and by 1900 there were nearly a score of such missions working in the London area. Additional missions had already been opened in Manchester (1870), Birmingham (1875), Glasgow (1878), Bristol (1873) and Dublin (1890).

The Edinburgh Medical Mission grew from a small Christian medical dispensary which had been opened by Dr. Handyside in the Cowgate area of the city. In 1861 this dispensary was taken over by the Edinburgh Medical Missionary Society, founded to support and prepare students in training for future service overseas. The students were introduced to some of the practical aspects of their future work. The E.M.M.S. mission hospitals at Nazareth and Damascus were also used for training and of these the Nazareth Hospital is still actively serving its community. A new building in Edinburgh — the Livingstone Dispensary — was erected in 1879 and the work continued as a direct Christian institution until 1952, when it was taken over by the University as a teaching centre for general practice.

THE MEDICAL WORK OF THE SALVATION ARMY

One of the major movements meeting the spiritual and social needs of the crowded cities was the Salvation Army, founded in 1865. In addition to its evangelistic and social work the Army also found it imperative to provide medical help for those who required it but could not afford or obtain it. In 1889 a home known as Ivy House was set up in Hackney for young women who, either through poverty or deception had been induced to turn to prostitution. Facilities were provided for the delivery of unmarried mothers when they found it difficult to gain admission elsewhere. A creche was also opened for mothers who had found work to do, but needed their babies to be cared for during working hours. In the first four years of its existence 500 women were delivered at Ivy House. The home soon began to train nurses and to develop a system of district midwifery, and during its first 18 years 506 nurses had been trained and 258 of them had obtained their Central Midwives Board Certificate. Figures published in 1981 gave a total of 3598 births at Ivy House itself and 7661 births attended in the homes of the district.

The Salvation Army carried the project for unmarried mothers overseas to Los Angeles (1890), Cape Town (1901), Winnipeg (1891), Melbourne (1897) and Christchurch, New Zealand (1882). The Mothers' Hospital in Clapton was opened in 1913, primarily for the unmarried, but at a later stage it also accepted married mothers. This hospital has developed into a specialist obstetric institution with high standards. (See also p. 158.)

CHILDREN'S HOSPITALS AND ORPHANAGES

Another area of need which attracted Christian action in the late 19th century was that of the children. That such attention was long overdue has been put beyond doubt by the genius of Dickens in his portrayal of the ordeals of childhood in *Oliver Twist, Bleak House* and the rest of his novels. He also highlighted the deplorable state of local hospital care for children by nurses who were 'habitually drunk, with easy-going, selfish indifference to their patients, and no knowledge or skill of nursing'! The necessity to plan special children's hospitals, with trained nurses, eventually caught the imagination of the public. In due course such havens were established in most of the major cities and some of them became world famous, as for example the Great Ormond Street Hospital in London. Many of these institutions have come to practise the highest standards in nursing and to offer the great advances which have been achieved in modern paediatrics and the related specialties such as orthopaedics.

DR BARNARDO'S HOMES

What appealed most of all to the emotions of the Christian public was the call to found homes for orphans, one of which will be featured here.

Thomas Barnardo was born in Dublin in 1845 and came to the London Hospital in order to prepare himself for work as a medical missionary in China. The early Christian influences in his life were from the Christian Brethren, but eventually he became an Anglican. As a student he carried on evangelistic work among children in the East End of London and it was this that opened his eyes to the need among homeless children. The story of Jim Jarvis who had no home to go to when Barnardo's Sunday School class had finished, and how he led Barnardo to a place where many other homeless children were sleeping under tarpaulins, is well known. With characteristic drive he stopped his medical training and founded the East End Juvenile Mission to help meet the situation. When 'Carrots', a destitute child, could not be admitted to the home because of lack of space, and was subsequently found dead from exposure and undernutrition, Barnardo laid down the principle of the ever open door. No destitute child was ever to be refused admission. Throughout this time he preached on Sundays in the Edinburgh Castle, a public house which he had bought and adapted for this purpose. He blandly assumed the title of 'doctor' although he was not fully qualified and he seems not to have gone into practice. When criticism was raised on this ground, he quietly went to Edinburgh and took a qualifying diploma.

Barnardo was a self-confident man, somewhat domineering and rather autocratic. When he saw a need he set about meeting it and later successfully appealed to the public for funds for his enterprise. No doubt it required a man of this type to achieve what he did. When he found the girls in his Barkingside home using coarse language, he began to build a village of cottages, with housemothers to bring to them some semblance of home life. He trained his boys for some craft, and the Watts naval school was part of this procedure. He embarked on an emigration scheme for sending his lads to Canada, and arranged for others to be boarded out with families. Darkin Williams has paid this tribute to him: 'Of many great men it might be said that religion tinged their lives. It would be inadequate to say that of Barnardo. His Christianity . . . not merely influenced his life, it was the propulsive power that dominated his career from start to finish. To try to explain Dr.Barnardo without his religion would be like trying to account for the fall of the apple without reference to the law of gravitation.' The man, with his great faith and vision, with all his drive and achievements, with his failings too, is vividly protrayed by his latest biographer, Gillian Wagner. Barnardo greatly influenced Lord Shaftesbury (p. 108)

While most of the homes for orphans were begun in the late 19th century, their major developments took place in the 20th. The appeals made by the leaders in the movement proved irresistible and many large and small institutions were started. Eventually most of the small, locally supported, homes in various cities joined with larger experienced organizations, such as Barnardo's, which had a wider national appeal. While Müller's Home in Bristol, Quarrier's near Glasgow and Fegan's in Kent continued on their strictly evangelical basis, the main national support became centred on the National Children's Homes (a Methodist foundation), the Church of England Children's Society and Dr. Barnardo's Homes. All of these societies have in recent times adapted more and more to present conditions, especially in seeking to place children into smaller 'family' units under acting 'parents', and also to ensure that, as far as possible, teenagers will be suitably and efficiently integrated into modern life.

TEMPERANCE MOVEMENTS

Another social evil (within the interests of Medicine) was excessive drinking and alcoholic addiction. The conditions in the mid-19th century, when wages were often paid to the workers at a public house, led to much increased drinking. Christian leaders began to act to reduce the trend, some aiming at securing moderation and others at total abstinence. As far back as the 18th century the Quaker doctors, for example Lettsom in 1791, regarded alcoholism as a disease and discussed prophylactic measures.

John Wesley in 1745 was among the first to exhort Christians not to buy, sell or drink alcoholic liquors except in necessity, that is, as a medicine. Towards the close of the 19th century the American evangelist, Dwight L. Moody, was similarly prominent in furthering the interests of self-discipline. North America vied with Britain in organizing societies to promote temperance. There was the American Temperance Society, the Rechabites, the Sons of Temperance, the Good Templars, the Blue Ribbon Movement and others. Though most temperance organizations were connected with branches of the Church, there were some which worked in neutral channels. Opinions differ as to the results achieved, though it is clear that there must have been a considerable reduction in drinking and considerable preventive influence. The United Kingdom Band of Hope Union — commenced by Mrs. Carlisle, widow of a Presbyterian minister, who aimed to influence younger children — had 26,000 local units and a membership of over 3 million in 1900. It appears, however, that some of the effective measures eventually came from legislation controlling the sale of alcoholic drinks, the times when they were available, the age of purchasers, and other conditions.

Two aspects of the temperance campaign which call for comment are the preventive measures taken and the pursuit of cure. The leaders in the movement were well aware that for working men in the evenings there was the lure of warmth, company and entertainment at the local public houses, and the continual temptation to drink. Beginning in 1854 in Dundee, where Lord Kinnaird established a coffee house at the suggestion of some working men, a movement swept across the country for funding 'coffee houses' in the cities and towns in which efforts were made to match 'the Trade' in everything except liquor.

It soon became evident that many cases of addiction would need long residential treatment and the various churches and the Salvation Army began to purchase suitable large houses as retreats. There were also government institutions and the National Institute for Inebriates. One of the most effective of the private ventures was Duxhurst Manor, Reigate, purchased in 1895 by Lady Henry Somerset. She was in advance of her time and clearly recognized addiction as a disease. Her regime slowly reduced the alcohol intake while her patients were kept occupied, given the run of the grounds and put to gardening and poultry farming. There was also a wise follow-up.

There is no doubt that at the beginning of this century the temperance movement had made a considerable impact, though not as much as the founders had hoped. The movement, however, had highlighted the extent and nature of the need, which aided the legislators who were moved to protect the wives and children. Conditions towards the end of the 20th century indicate that a renewed effort will be needed to combat the effects of addiction to alcohol.

THE BLIND AND THE DEAF

The scope of the reforms attempted by the 19th century Evangelicals included attention to the plight of the blind and deaf. The leaders first called the attention of the public to the extent of the problem and then began to take remedial action long before state legislation, such as the Elementary Education: Blind and Deaf Children Act of 1893, came into force. It took some time before there was agreement on the best aims and methods, but eventually several nationwide societies emerged which made a real impression and achieved satisfactory standards of service.

The first traceable steps in aid for the blind were to be found in the 1780s in Paris, where Valentin Hauy had opened schools for the blind. In England these were imitated by Edward Rushton's Liverpool School for the Blind (1791), by the Quakers in Bristol (1793) where their school grew into the Royal School of Industry for the Blind, and (as a memorial to William Wilberforce) the Yorkshire School for the Blind.

Not, however, until 1868 were fuller and more efficient steps taken with an adequate plan for teaching the blind to read and to train them for future remunerative work. An evangelical churchman and general practitioner, Dr. Thomas Rhodes Armitage, began to find that he was losing his own sight. As a student he had seen the work done for the blind in Germany and France. He decided to give up his medical practice and devote his remaining years to promoting education for young blind persons. His wife devoted her attention to the elderly blind. In 1868 they founded a society for 'Promoting the Education and Employment of the Blind', which eventually developed into the Royal National Institute for the Blind.

It was Dr. and Mrs. Armitage who painstakingly searched everywhere for the best form of embossed script to enable the blind to read and who eventually chose and promoted Braille on a world scale. Other effective steps followed. For example, it was Dr. Armitage who prevailed on the American musician Francis Campbell to stay with him in England and help to organize the Royal Normal College for the Blind. Campbell embossed the music so that the blind could be trained as organists and piano tuners. By 1885 the College had taught 170 trainees to earn their living by piano tuning and acting as organists. Numerous other services were to follow to meet a variety of needs as, for example, the Sunshine Homes for Blind Babies.

A similar series of activities was designed to meet the needs of the deaf. These also began in small local societies which eventually flowed together into national societies with increased standards and efficiency. The essential steps from the first beginnings to a system of education and employment for the deaf are owed to two Evangelicals, Thomas Arnold (Minister of Doddridge Chapel, Nottingham) and William Stainer (a teacher). They persevered with plans for educating the deaf in special classes at ordinary schools and then (where parents had difficulty in taking and fetching) in residential Stainer Homes. Eventually the fully developed Royal National Institute for the Deaf (1911) brought the various elements together and helped to raise the services to acceptable modern standards.

OTHER FORMS OF HANDICAP

Space precludes consideration of the many other forms of medical and sociological problems which were confronted by these tireless Christian voluntary societies before the state intervened with major legislation such as its Health Insurance Acts and other measures which finally culminated in the National Health Insurance Act of 1946. The total in gifts of money, time and skills on the part of the Christian public and the self-sacrifice of the army of voluntary workers is beyond computation. It represented an immense and indispensable supplement to the work of the medical and nursing professions at a time of great expansion. It is easy for critics with the advantage of hindsight and the easier personal circumstances of today to deprecate the foibles of some of our forefathers and to pronounce confidently what they *ought* to have done! The total of what *was* done remains a magnificent monument to their diligent and undaunted charity.

It should be added here that there are records of similar feats of Christian charity in the various other Protestant and Roman Catholic regions of the world. Voluntary giving and voluntary service have been seen on a similarly vast scale, especially in Germany, Scandinavia, Holland and North America. Each of these countries has added its quota to the impressive whole.

THE MODERN HOSPICE MOVEMENT

In recent years Christian initiative in Britain has returned to one of the strong points of the Church of the third and fourth centuries. A new hospice movement has come into being to provide as peaceful an environment as possible for those in their terminal illness. The concept of a hospice is not only directed to provide for specialized nursing, but also to offer a total environment of Christian love and support.

The movement began in 1905 when the Sisters of Charity from Ireland founded St. Joseph's Hospice in Hackney, East London. Their work has grown until, in recent years, it can claim that annually some 600 cancer patients received 'pain control and final comforts'. As a result of what she saw while working at St. Joseph's, Dame Cicely Saunders founded St. Christopher's Hospice at Sydenham, South London, in 1967. This has served as a model not only in its whole Christian approach to the problem of terminal illness, but also in the residential interdisciplinary courses which it offers for nurses and medical and theological students. The success of St. Joseph's and St. Christopher's stimulated the growth of a widespread movement which has resulted in a number of hospices being opened, such as St. Anne's, Manchester and St. Francis's, Romford. The movement has spread to the Continent and to North America.

Dr. R. W. Luxton, a retired Manchester physician, has highlighted the aim of these institutions by suggesting that 'in the hospice the centre of interest has shifted from the disease to the patient, from the pathology to the person'. The patient feels part of the teamwork of the treatment and is finally enabled to take leave of the world with dignity and serenity. It is particularly important that the spiritual aspect of the hospice movement should be retained. One of the doctor founders of another hospice writes in his annual report: 'The early units had such ideals, but they seem sadly lacking in some of newer ones. Without that "extra dimension" we are doing little more than creating yet another specialty. The dead hand of secularization down the years has so often overlooked the springs from which have sprung the essential good.'

CHAPTER 13

THE SPREAD OF WESTERN MEDICINE

By
GORDON A. D. LAVY
Formerly on the staff of the Mengo Hospital, Uganda

IT might be expected that the development of Medicine in the West would sooner or later result in the benefits diffusing to less advanced regions. However, several factors tended, initially at least, to impede such a spread: limited communication, cultural barriers, suspicion of the new, inertia and the inevitable lack of money and messengers. On the other hand the great need and the great benefits often attainable with fairly simple measures and limited outlay encouraged many to seek opportunities to share the fruit of medical advance with the multitude whose need was (and still is) so great.

Neither the state of medical knowledge, even at its best, nor the available means of communication allowed much movement before the end of the 18th century. Even then Africa and Asia were slow to benefit, for while various organizations, such as the East India Company, employed doctors to look after their own staff, there was little attempt to offer aid to the indigenous population. Some doctors, no doubt, would have sought to express their compassion in a practical way, but would equally certainly have been discouraged by the overwhelming volume of the need and their own pathetically inadequate resources.

When a change came, it was largely the influence of Christianity that brought the idea of care and so of practical help for those in such need in the native communities. Thus it was usually, if not always, through missionary activities that medical help began to be introduced.

THE FIRST MEDICAL MISSIONARIES

One of the earliest, if not the first, doctor to carry his knowledge to the East was a German Lutheran, Kaspar Gottlieb Schlegemilch who went as a medical missionary to India in 1730 under joint Danish and German auspices. Sadly, he died within a month of reaching Madras. Later in the 18th century John Thomas, originally a medical officer with the East India

Company, went out from England in 1793 with the Baptist Missionary Society. Thomas worked for a while with William Carey and was highly regarded for his medical skill. Among the first Protestant doctors to go to Africa as a missionary was J. van der Kemp in 1799.

The first American medical missionary seems to have been Dr. John Scudder who went to Ceylon (now Sri Lanka) in 1819. There can have been few families in which the missionary tradition became established to such an extent for, in the next three generations, 32 members of the Scudder family gave 1500 years of service to India.

Even in the 19th century, however, missionary societies did not always give very much priority to medical work. They believed that attention to such needs was a diversion from preaching the gospel and an unjustified economic strain on their slender resources. Thus, even by 1850, there were only some 12 to 15 medical missionaries in all the non-Christian world. So, when Peter Parker went to China in 1834 under the American Board of Commissioners for Foreign Missions, he went to a virgin field so far as Western Medicine was concerned. His reputation rapidly spread beyond Canton where he started what was primarily an ophthalmic hospital in 1835. While operating on a wide range of conditions his work in ophthalmology came to be in particular demand. It was said that 'Dr. Parker opened the gates of China with a lancet when European cannon could not heave a single bar'.

Of equal, or greater, importance than his clinical work was his training of Chinese assistants. In 1845 he had five students under regular instruction. A man of enormous energy and imagination, he found time to foster diplomatic relations between China and the U.S.A. When he died in 1888 at the age of 83 his contributions to the developing world included being the first medical missionary to China, the first to found a modern hospital in the Far East, the first to use an anaesthetic there and the first to start medical education under Christian auspices. In addition to all this, during a visit to Edinburgh he had been instrumental in the founding of the Edinburgh Medical Missionary Society (see p. 147) under the presidency of John Abercrombie, who had already in 1841 sponsored the Edinburgh Association for sending Medical Aid to Foreign Countries.

While David Livingstone is chiefly remembered as an explorer, his original resolve was 'to devote my life to the alleviation of human misery', and he went to Southern Africa as a medical missionary in 1841. Towards the end of his life he wrote, 'If the good Lord above gives me strength and influence to complete the task in spite of everything, I shall not grudge my hunger and toils. Above all, if He permits me to put a stop to the enormous evils of this inland slave trade I shall bless His name with all my heart. The Nile sources are valuable to me only as a means of opening my mouth with power among men.' When he died in 1873 he had opened the door of Africa and paved the way for the doctor as well as the preacher and trader.

The pioneer work of David Livingstone in South Africa, Bechuanaland (Botswana), Nyasaland (Malawi), the Rhodesias (Zambia and Zimbabwe), Congo (Zaire) and Tanganyika (Tanzania) was continued by a succession of Christian doctors who established missions and hospitals in various parts of these countries. This process has continued in the 20th century and Christian doctors and nurses have been instrumental in building up a health service for black Southern African peoples aided by provincial and central governments. It was the missions, also, that were the first to train African nurses and midwives who in turn put into practice in their own homes and environments the principles of good hygiene and nutrition which they had learned. The contribution of medical missionaries in Southern and Central Africa was probably one of the largest in the world.

THE OPENING OF THE THIRD WORLD

So, in the second half of the 19th century, Africa became an example of the gradual diffusion of Western medicine to the under-developed parts of the world. This occurred not only as a result of more medically orientated policies of the great missionary societies, but also by the development of medical services under the colonial system, especially within the British Empire. Nationals of many European countries played a part in this expansion. Perhaps the best known figure was that remarkable genius, Albert Schweitzer, whose mission hospital at Lambarene in West Africa became one of the most widely known medical missionary enterprises. Undoubtedly this was largely due to the interest attaching to the doctor himself. For here was a man who, with enormous academic distinction in theology, music and medicine, nevertheless buried himself in remote forest country in Gabon for the sake of the gospel. But there were many others, less publicized, who went out with the same motive.

In East Africa, Albert Cook, sent by the Church Missionary Society, founded Mengo Hospital just outside Kampala in Uganda in 1897. A trained eye and an acute mind brought not only aid to many sufferers but a steadily increasing knowledge of local diseases. In 1901, with his brother, J. H. Cook, he first recognized sleeping sickness in the try-panosomiasis epidemic of Uganda. His records are still a fruitful and accurate source of information. He is representative of many who at this period were taking Western medical knowledge to the ends of the earth, and not only applying it, but seeking to train the local inhabitants to apply it themselves. His knighthood in 1932 was a recognition of his work both as a practising doctor and as a teacher.

The last half of the 19th century and the first part of the 20th saw a very vigorous growth of Christian medical activity in Africa and Asia. Between 1850 and 1950 more than 1500 British doctors went to Christian medical institutions in the developing countries, and many also went from Scandinavian, German, Dutch and American missionary organizations. Among these were John Kerr and William Wanless who both served with the American Presbyterian Missionary Society, the former in China where he was responsible for preparing Chinese textbooks of medicine, and the latter in India where he founded the hospital and medical school at Miraj which has been described as 'one of the finest missionary institutions in India'. Another pioneer was Rudolph Fisch, a Swiss medical missionary in Ghana. He produced a book on tropical medicine based on his experience. Among the church-related hospitals, the two largest international networks are those of the Roman Catholic Church and the Salvation Army.

The Salvation Army's medical work overseas began in India when Harry Andrews, a lad in his late teens, went with his adoptive parents to the extreme south of the country. At first he provided first aid treatment, including dental extractions and suturing, to the needy people of the area, but in 1893 he extended the work by opening a primitive dispensary to which patients came for treatment from many miles around. He returned to England to take a dresser's course at a London hospital and, on returning to India in 1896, set up a full-scale dispensary which was financed through the gift of a friend. From this small beginning there developed the first Salvation Army mission hospital, the Catherine Booth Hospital at Nagercoil. Andrews later set up the Emery Hospital at Amand, Gujarat, and in 1912 the Thomas Emery Hospital in North India. Meanwhile, he had been sent to study medicine in the U.S.A. where he eventually qualified. He was seconded to the military some years afterwards and in 1919 he was killed in action on the northwest frontier while rescuing wounded soldiers under fire. For this he was awarded the V.C. posthumously — the last doctor to receive this distinction.

During the first half of the 20th century there was an expansion of government sponsored medical services in the developing world. Since the end of World War II this has been followed by a gradual withdrawal of the missionary agencies from major medical commitments. This has happened largely because of rapidly increasing costs, though sometimes the problem has been eased by the acceptance by government of the financial burden of the hospital services. But while the hospital-based facilities may be passing to official agencies, there remain great opportunities for Christian initiative in other directions such as primary care and health education which need less sophisticated and expensive means.

SOLVING TROPICAL DISEASES

While many disorders of the Western world find their counterpart in the developing areas, some conditions are confined to particular regions. Patient investigation and research on the spot is needed before the cause can be found and suitable methods of treatment or prevention evolved.

Often the initiatives in the investigation, treatment and prophylaxis of tropical diseases were first undertaken by medical officers serving with the armed forces of the colonial powers — French, Portuguese, British, Dutch and German. But often, perhaps because they have been earlier at the frontiers in the field, mission doctors have also been in the forefront of such endeavours. It may be, of course, that after initial observations had been made, more sophisticated research was required which, because of time, cost and equipment, could not be undertaken on the spot. But to start the search was an essential step. The recognition of sleeping sickness in Uganda by the brothers Cook has already been mentioned. Early observations suggested *Filaria perstans* as a possible cause, a view supported by no lesser authority than Patrick Manson. Though disproved eventually, the search for, and discovery of, the role of the trypanosome and the tsetse fly was sparked off by a communication published by the Cook brothers. It was this that stirred Manson into pressing for a commission to investigate the outbreak.

The often prolonged interval between the recognition of a particular problem and its solution presents a tremendous opportunity for the Christian doctor to exhibit loving care and practical help. This is well illustrated by the continuing battle with the scourge of leprosy. Since the discovery of the casual agent, *Mycobacterium leprae,* by the Norwegian

Gerard Henrik Armauer Hansen, a search for curative agents has continued with gradually increasing success. But in the earlier years, when little could be done in this respect, the social and physical miseries of the sufferers stirred medical missionaries and others into relief measures. Dr. and Mrs. E. G. Horder of the Church Missionary Society started the first modern leprosy hospital at Pakhoi in China at the end of the 19th century. Since then many other workers have devoted themselves to giving help with the medical and social problems of the disease in many parts of the world. High in any list must come the names of Christian missionaries such as Ernest Muir and Robert Cochrane in South India, Frank Davey in Nigeria, Leonard Sharp on his island settlement in Lake Bunyoni in Uganda, Duncan Main in Hong Kong, and more recently Stanley Browne with a roving commission to offer his vast experience in counsel and encouragement on a world-wide basis. Even when arrested or cured, leprosy often leaves gross deformities both cosmetically and functionally. Paul Brand, working at the Vellore Christian Medical College in South India, pioneered much work in restoring function to arms and legs by surgical means.

Sometimes a particular problem demands virtually all the attention of the individual doctor. Leprosy is one such; another is blindness. Here, too, the problem is a huge one. The causes are many. Trachoma is one of a number of diseases which are largely the result of poor hygiene, dust and malnutrition, and its control must depend on dealing with these causes. Other disorders, such as cataract, are more immediately amenable to surgery.

It was to this field that Henry Holland devoted the greater part of his life in Quetta on the northwest frontier of the subcontinent of India. One of the major problems was the sheer numbers involved. He and his team would sometimes tackle 180 eye operations a day and the patients would be laid in rows to recover as he moved on to the next clinic centre. He is said to have completed over 40,000 operations for cataract — the last at the age of 81. Sir Henry, as he became, was a legend in his own lifetime and 'retired' at least twice before he died aged 90. Similarly J. M. Macphail at the Free Church of Scotland's Bamdah Mission Hospital in Bihar is reputed to have operated on more ophthalmic cases in one year than were completed by a dozen surgeons at Moorfields Hospital, London, in seven or eight years. His work was continued by his son, R. M. Macphail.

Sometimes the attack on disease may take other than purely medical forms. (Sir) Wilfred Grenfell, who went as a medical missionary to Labrador, saw the need for economic help for the Eskimos and put his understanding into action by starting saw mills to make use of the natural resources, setting up farms to cultivate the silver fox and by importing reindeer, as well as establishing a cooperative to aid in the marketing of fish. The economic wellbeing of people, in so far as it involves their physical and mental wellbeing, becomes one of the wider concerns of the doctor. It may involve him in the manipulation of the environment!

Similarly one prong in the advance against tuberculosis and some other diseases involves economic factors — the removal of poor living conditions, inadequate hygiene, malnutrition and ignorance. This opens vistas of preventive medicine. Here is a vast, largely untouched, field where the trust and confidence engendered by patient, disinterested love and compassion (that should be the hallmark of Christian missionary enterprise) can reap a harvest by fostering cooperation in campaigns to combat a particular local problem. Such projects may include schemes for mass inoculation and efforts to change long established traditions which may be dangerous. One example of the latter is the use in some parts of Uganda of 'native medicine', which is a powerful oxytocic drug used to stimulate the onset of labour and which may be disastrous in the presence of disproportion. Another is the application of dung as a dressing for the child's umbilicus following birth. All too often tetanus ensues. Such deeply ingrained customs are difficult to break, but reinforcement of the truth built up over the years by faithful medical missionaries and mission nurses and others is the strongest weapon in the fight. Their names may not be recorded, but the debt owed to them by succeeding generations is very great.

By no means all the disease of the Third World is peculiar to it, and many problems are common to all the continents. At Neyyoor in South India S. H. Pugh pioneered work on peptic ulcer and its surgical management. His work was continued by Howard Somervell and Ian Orr and in 1936 they published the results of 2500 cases with a mortality of only just over 2%.

IN OTHER SERVICES

Christian doctors in the developing countries have not always worked in the framework of medical missions; many have been in the Armed or Government services. Walter Reed was the son of an American Methodist minister and was himself an active Christian. He had been the youngest student to qualify in Medicine at Virginia University. He entered the Army Medical Service and was engaged in postgraduate study in bacteriology in Welch's department at the Johns Hopkins when the call of duty induced him to volunteer for work with the Yellow Fever Commission in Havana, which had been set up to investigate an outbreak of the disease among American soldiers stationed in Cuba.

One of the team had noted that direct contact with a victim was frequently not followed by infection and that there was always an interval before the disease spread to others. These circumstances led Reed to postulate a vector, probably an insect. In due course the *Aedes aegypti* was incriminated and Reed's efforts were devoted to controlling the breeding grounds which were always near human habitation. His easy personality and the avoidance of compulsion (though within his powers) enabled him to get the trust and cooperation of the local population. Within a year Havana was cleared of yellow fever. It is ironic that he should have died from appendicitis soon after his work was finished while two of his colleagues, who allowed themselves to be bitten by suspect mosquitoes, contracted yellow fever, and one of them died. A friend said of him, 'When his great work was accomplished the happiness which filled his soul was entirely for the suffering he would spare humanity. He rejoiced that he had not lived in vain and that God had seen fit to make him an instrument of good.'

Ronald Ross, with a Christian background, went out to find the carrier of the malarial organism when he was a young doctor in the Indian army. In the course of his work he examined many mosquitoes, looking for the parasite. One evening he seemed about to have another fruitless and frustrating session. He had almost finished when, looking at the stomach tissues of the last mosquito of the batch, he found the parasite and the role of the *anopheles* mosquito was finally beyond question. It was the 20th August 1897. The great discovery had been made, and in a letter to his wife Ross penned verses giving praise to God, for he foresaw what enormous benefits the control of malaria would confer on millions yet unborn.

In the 1960s Denis Burkitt, a Christian surgeon in the Colonial Service working in Uganda, patiently followed clues leading to the identification of the vector and the casual organism of the tumour now known by his name. Since then chemotherapy has made a dramatic change in the outlook of this type of childhood malignancy.

MEDICAL EDUCATION

While initially help from outside may be essential, long-term progress in medical care must aim at being self-supporting in money, materials and manpower. And the latter, among other things, means medical schools and the training of the indigenous doctor. Only so can the numbers needed be obtained. They will also have the immense advantage that doctor and patient will share a common language, customs and background. It follows that the ultimate aim of the expatriate doctor, whether missionary or otherwise, is to make himself redundant. The need for this has also been emphasized by the currently rising tide of nationalism and the spread of Communism.

The value of training local individuals was early realized. It has already been mentioned that Peter Parker had a number of Chinese assistants undergoing training as early as the 1840s. Subsequently many missionary doctors saw that the benefit they brought could be more widely spread if a number of individuals were taught a few simple procedures and were then sent out to surrounding villages from the main base.

In 1935 (Sir) Clement Chesterman working with the Baptist Missionary Society at Yakusu Hospital on the Congo River started to train native medical assistants to serve the surrounding forest villages. The project was taken up in 1936 by the newly arrived Stanley G. Browne, who developed the three year curriculum, supplemented by practical courses at rural centres and followed by periodic refresher courses. The result was welcomed and recognized by the (then) Belgian Colonial Government. Eventually Stanley Browne completed the training of over 300 *infirmiers* (and a number of women *infirmières* for midwifery) and established 18 rural medical centres served by them. *Infirmiers* were also supplied to 15 other Protestant Missions in Zaire.

The provision of a full medical course remains a much larger undertaking. It requires vision, energy and courage, perhaps beyond the average, to see through the enormous difficulties and then press on undaunted. Those who succeed stand out as being outside the common mould. The debt to them of succeeding generations is immeasurable.

In 1893 a young American, Oliver Avison, who founded Severance Union Medical College in Seoul, was told that he was a fool to think he could have much effect on the millions in Korea. His response was to say that while he could not care for many himself, he could train ten Korean doctors. In the event he trained many more. This medical school was the first institution founded under Christian auspices in the Far East. From China, a little earlier, Fang Wu had gone to Edinburgh for medical training and had returned to China in 1887, supported by the London Missionary Society. He achieved a great professional reputation and was followed by others. But such an enterprise, valuable as it was, could not provide for the full medical needs of China, perhaps representing 20% of the world's population. By the time of the Communist take-over in China six medical schools had been started by Christian endeavour, with another in Manchuria. In 1944 the then Director General of the National Health Department of China said this: 'It is fitting that warmest thanks and highest tribute be paid to the Christian medical services, in all forms, for the fundamentally important part they have played and continue to play in the development of modern medical practice in China.' And it looks as if the door, closed with the Communist take-over, may be edging open again.

In India medical training in some of the universities had started in the first half of the 19th century under the British Raj. But the need, as ever, outstripped supply and three Christian medical schools were started in order to respond to the continuing shortage and to make a distinctive Christian contribution.

In 1894 Edith Brown founded Ludhiana Medical College in North India for women students. In 1897 William Wanless opened Miraj for men; and in South India in 1918 Ida Scudder started medical training at the hospital she had opened at Vellore. She was a member of the American Scudder family, already mentioned, whose score in terms of number of members and years served must be a record in overseas missionary endeavour. Dr. Ida opened her original one bed unit in 1900, the year after she qualified. In 1909 a school of nursing was started. In 1942 the Indian Government decided that all medical training should be of university degree standard and to this end the Miraj medical school, after much heart-searching, was closed and amalgamated with Vellore. In 1950 there came affiliation with Madras University, but first and foremost Vellore remained a Christian institution and was acknowledged to be among the best of the medical colleges in Asia. Such was the view of Gandhi. By 1950 it was reporting an annual total of over 5000 operations. Miraj (the hospital) was linked in 1962 with a newly established medical college in the State of Maharashtra, but the Christian status of the hospital was retained.

In East Africa Albert Cook had gone to Uganda under the Church Missionary Society in 1896. He and his party walked the 850 miles from Mombasa, a journey which took nearly three months. They arrived at the capital, Kampala, in February 1897 and within three days Cook had started work. A 12 bed hospital was opened, soon to be expanded because of pressing need. In spite of the help of his brother Jack, the need for African assistants became obvious. He therefore started a course for medical assistants in 1917. This initial venture, as time went by, was handed over to the Government and expanded into the present medical school of the university of Makerere. Until the independence of the East African territories this was the only such school serving Uganda, Kenya and Tanzania.

A very happy situation arises when after medical training elsewhere, a man returns as a 'missionary' to his own country. Such occurred with Fang Wu, and such occurred again when Francis Akanu Ibiam, who graduated in medicine from St. Andrews in 1936, returned to Nigeria under the auspices of the Church of Scotland. He served at Itu and Calabar, opening his own mission hospital at Abiriba and was a medical missionary for 20 years. A man of distinction, he became civil governor of the Eastern Region of Nigeria in 1960. Previous to that, as chairman of the University Council at Ibadan he did much to inspire the students during his tenure of office. A relatively small group of medical men and women have been called to do great work both on an individual basis and as statesman with a wider influence on succeeding generations. Of such a group Ibiam was one.

A striking example of the industrious pioneer work accomplished by many of the first medical missionaries is presented by the life of Robert Laws of Aberdeen. He qualified first in theology and then, by part-time study, in Medicine. He was sent in 1875 by the Free Church of Scotland mission to Livingstonia as leader and medical officer at Cape Maclear. In 1876 he introduced chloroform to Nyasaland (Malawi), using it to remove a cystic tumour from an eye. He established stations at Bandawe (1881) and at Livingstonia, a healthier hill site at the northern end of the lake (1894). He regarded evangelism, industrial training and medical work as all part of the field's development, and he developed the Overtoun Institute (on the model of James Stewart's Lovedale Institute in S. Africa) to train artisans and clerks. Between 1901 and 1905 13 African hospitals were built, and in 1911 the David Gordon Memorial Hospital was opened. It had the first X-ray unit in the country and became a key training hospital. Laws was an unofficial member of the Nyasaland Legislative Assembly 1912-1916.

Laws's senior colleague, the remarkably able James Stewart of Glasgow, was also medically qualified. Although the influence of the Lovedale Missionary Institute, of which he became principal in 1870, was largely religious, educational and industrial, at the centre of the buildings was an up-to-date hospital. Stewart was a pioneer in medical missions.

He was the first to found a rural hospital in native Africa, to start the training of nurses and hospital assistants, and to lay the foundations for a developing medical school.

A number of other medical schools in various parts of the world, not now specifically Christian, were originally started as church based institutions. One such is that associated with the American University of Beirut in the Lebanon; another is the Union Medical College in Peking, founded in 1900 by Thomas Cochrane of the London Missionary Society. By the time of the Japanese invasion of China in the 1930s five other Christian medical schools had been founded, including one at Mukden. Here Dugald Christie under the United Presbyterian Church pioneered a medical school which in due course was training 200 students. Christie was also active in halting the epidemics of plague in Manchuria in 1910 and 1911.

Today the rapidly increasing cost of medical training, and indeed of hospitals, has meant that missionary bodies have been unable to continue on the same scale in these fields, certainly without government support. While in some cases this has been generously given and the specifically Christian initiatives have been maintained, in the main the larger schemes have been taken over by the Government authorities. Missionary medical enterprise has had to be channelled into other fields. The emphasis now, therefore, is put more on areas where the cover is thinnest – outside the larger centres – and also on preventative work and the training of health workers in the community. It is still education in fact, but this time of the ordinary citizen rather than of the professional.

This sort of work is not dramatic and does not produce the pioneer heroes of the past, but it is just as vital and potentially of longer lasting value. Christian doctors have been in the forefront of preventive medicine and ground-roots education. Such work is unremitting, not overgenerous in its visible rewards, and sometimes plain discouraging, but it is more than worth while. Patience, love and perseverance are still the essential qualifications.

SOME IMPORTANT STATISTICS

Medical Missions at Home and Abroad, the journal of the Medical Missionary Association of London, published in 1889 a list of societies which were together supporting 128 British doctors who were serving overseas. World figures, for all Protestant Missions, first became available in 1925 and were given in the *World Missionary Atlas* published by the Conference of Missionary Societies, Edinburgh House. The Atlas marked the sites on the maps where mission stations existed and statistics were attached.

The 1925 Atlas gave the total number of missionary doctors, who qualified in Europe or North America, as 1154. To these were to be added another 614 nationals, who had qualified as doctors in their own countries. This brought the total of doctors to 1768. Many of the latter were trained in the Christian Medical Colleges of which there were 19 providing a full medical course and, at the time, they had an indigenous medical student membership of 914. In addition to the provision for medical students, there were 66 training schools for nurses in which 1932 nurses were following a full nurses' training. On the staffs of these hospitals were 1008 qualified nurses, who were missionaries, and 5458 indigenous men and women medical 'assistants' in various stages of nurses' training.

In the year 1963 the Missionary Research Library of New York gave similar statistics in the *Directory of Protestant Church-Related Hospitals,* outside of Europe and North America. In that year there were 1231 Christian Hospitals and other institutions such as maternity hospitals and leprosaria. Staffing these hospitals were 828 qualified doctors who were supported by Missionary Societies and 1317 medical qualified colleagues who qualified in their own countries, giving a total of 2145 doctors. Serving with them were 1321 qualified nurses from overseas and 6928 indigenous nurses, most of the latter having been trained in their own countries. (It is believed that accurate figures would be considerably in excess of the figures given above, which were based on the returns received. No details were received from some of the mission hospitals.)

For the past hundred years there have been strong medical units sent to parts of Asia and Africa by the Lutheran Churches of Germany, Scandinavia and North America. During the last twenty years some 75 doctors and 250 nurses have been sent from Germany to the Christian hospitals in the developing countries. Support in the form of drugs and surgical equipment are all channelled through the Deutches Institut für Ärztliche Mission, which also maintains its Hospital for Tropical Diseases at Tübingen.

The two British societies, which came into being in the 19th century to increase the number of doctors serving in the Christian hospitals and tribal areas overseas, are still active though the conditions have changed. The Edinburgh Medical Missionary Society (1841) has helped over 420 missionary candidates to qualify as doctors and the Medical Missionary Association, London (1878) has similarly assisted some 300 more. Like Edinburgh, each of the London teaching hospitals has given its quota of medicals to the Christian missions (and also to the former Indian Medical Service and other Government medical services). In 1980 the Christian Union of the Royal Free Hospital Medical School (which until after World War II trained only women students) issued a brochure with a list of 233 women doctors who from that hospital alone have served mostly in the Christian mission hospitals.

For the centuries after the Reformation this book has concentrated on the work in the Protestant medical circles. It must, however, be remembered that in more recent years the agencies of the Roman Catholic Church have similarly given extensive service throughout the world. Complete statistics do not appear to be available, but mention of only two of the relevant Orders will give some impression of the scope of what has been done. The Order of the Sisters of Mary (founded in 1939 at Drogheda, Eire) had in 1967 sent 41 doctors, 2 dentists, 15 sister-tutors and 159 nurses. They had treated 946,647 patients, of which 131,647 were maternity cases and 13,909 sufferers from leprosy. Similarly in 1981 the Medical Mission Sisters (Anna Dergel's Foundation), based on Rome, had a total of 697 doctors serving overseas.

CHAPTER 14

EPILOGUE

THE aim of the writers of these chapters has been historical. They have sought to put on record the chief contributions made by Christians to Western Medicine. At several points they have thought it relevant also to illustrate the extent to which Christianity as a whole has proved a major and beneficent ally to the science of healing, which has now grown to world proportions. They are aware, however, that the study has several limitations and these call for explanation.

First, in no way has it been intended to imply that Christians have always been in the vanguard of progress and have not made their mistakes. In the Dark and Middle Ages priest-medicine failed to free itself from some of the mistaken traditions received from antiquity and the superstititions and prejudices of their time. The Church's ban on the dissection of the human body and on the priests' use of a scalpel undoubtedly delayed advances in surgery. Similarly, fear of the Inquisition retarded many a potential experiment and slowed progress in other branches of Medicine. Even in modern times ecclesiastical conservatism has been mistaken for the demands of true Christian ethics. On balance, however, and certainly from the time of the Reformation, the main trend has been in the right direction.

Secondly, there has been no desire to overlook, or underestimate, the many advances made by those of other religions or philosophies. At the outset attention was drawn to the two large volumes of *The Jews in Medicine* and, in the 19th and 20th centuries, especially in Germany and the United States, many crucial discoveries came from members of that race. Similarly, leading Arab doctors of the early Middle Ages added significantly to the borrowed traditions of the West before these were later returned to Europe through Salerno and Montpellier. Then, during the last 100 years, many of the outstanding discoveries which have completely transformed Medicine were the work of scientific humanists.

Then, several reasons have tended to bring the examples in most of the chapters to a halt early in the 20th century. The chief of these has been that in modern times in all branches of science it has become more difficult to assign credit to the individuals to whom it is due. In place of the gifted individual medical adviser (or the lone research worker) there is now in support a team of highly trained specialists. With the increased technical complexities in diagnosis, treatment and total care, the medical services to the public and scientific advances in the specialties became a corporate rather than an individual activity. Also, with the great increase of the state's economic and administrative involvement in the doctor-patient relationship and in the work of the hospital laboratory, the group involvement eclipses the individual.

A CENTURIES OLD TRADITION

In the light of the facts of medical history we would suggest that Christianity and individual Christians have, over the years, made a major contribution to the rise and world spread of Western Medicine. To the Christians belongs the credit of raising the social status and treatment of sick and handicapped persons in early times. To them also belongs the credit, from the fourth century down to the 19th or 20th, of the voluntary financing of the greater number of hospices, general hospitals and specialist hospitals for the sick and various types of handicapped. From its very size and complexity, the full story may never be fully told. In addition to this, it was the Churches which produced by far the greater number of the nurses and other personnel to staff these hospitals.

There have been numerous other points where Christians have been in the vanguard or strongly represented among those physicians and other practitioners who, sometimes in the face of misunderstanding and public criticism, have achieved key advances in medicine or surgery. They have borne their fair share in the progress of medical education and medical writing. Many have been pioneers and served a key role in the development of medical ethics. They are needed all the more in the acute problems of today where 'feasibility' could easily become the arbiter of what is right.

Then, the Christian religion has an important bearing on several areas of practice, for example the necessity of truth. If he follows the inner logic of his own religion, the Christian who claims to obey the God of truth is necessarily required to speak and act it. Truth is also closely related to justice. The inner thrust of the Christian's religion requires justice (in the form of love) for his 'neighbour' the patient. As the prophet reminds us: 'And what does the Lord require of you but to do justly, and to love mercy, and to walk humbly with your God' (Micah 6:8).

Christians have also been among the pioneers of immunology, public health and preventive medicine. Then, in the 19th and 20th centuries, with medical missions and Christian hospitals, they were in the vanguard of those who carried Western Medicine across the world.

The evidence is particularly strong in the biographies of those responsible for achieving higher standards in Medicine, Nursing and related professions. Many dedicated women entered on their nursing careers with a deep sense of vocation. Memoirs of a number of the great Matrons and Sister-Tutors of well-known teaching hospitals reveal the inspiration and quiet confidence which they derived from their Christian faith. Medicine's debt to them, and those similarly motivated in more lowly positions, is indeed very great. Nor must we forget the clergy and Free Church ministers who kept the ideal of such professions before their young people, nor the hospital chaplains who have conscientiously pursued their difficult and often thankless tasks.

When these traditional sources of recruitment and inspiration grow less, or are missing, the differences can be keenly felt, though the reason for it may remain unrecognized. An article in the *British Medical Journal* (February 1981) commented: 'As the influence of the Church declines until its effect is negligible, as fewer and fewer people are encouraged to, or are willing to, take responsibility . . . a general lowering of standards seems inevitable.' It was no accident that the morale in the medical, nursing and all related professions was at its highest in the late 19th and early 20th centuries when the Christian Churches and Christian influence were at their peak.

MOTIVATION

One of the commonest misunderstandings of observers unfamiliar with the Christian religion is to imagine that its practice is subject to a set of rules for following what (to them) is an impossible ideal. It is here that the history of the Christian influence in Medicine should have a moral. The dynamic force which energizes the Christian's life in the pursuit of his ideal is personal. Obedience to Christ, prompted in the heart of the believer by the Holy Spirit, is motivated by *gratitude* — gratitude for what Christ *has done* for him — and a return of love to God for God's prior love to him. This form of divine love is the nerve centre of Christian ethics and the force which overrides circumstances and difficulties and keeps the Christian at his post.

CHRISTIAN MEN IN MEDICINE

This issue, as applied to Medicine, has been well described by Douglas Jackson, formerly a surgeon on the Burns Unit of the Birmingham Accident Hospital, in a paper for medical students. He writes: 'The idea that a Christian doctor in a scientific age will practise technical medicine in a way which is different from (or even better than) a non-Christian doctor is a popular misconception. There is a self-evident distinction between good medicine and bad, but to see a difference between Christian medicine and non-Christian medicine is an illusion. In fact, as we all know, many non-Christian doctors are better than many Christian doctors at their job because they are more gifted, wiser, stronger or more hardworking; they may have deeper insights or be more warm-hearted and humane. Spiritual regeneration does not add to a man's physical propensities. His brain and capacities are not elevated out of the second class into those of the first class or genius.'

'If we return to the question, then, "does being a Christian make no difference?", the answer is that it makes no difference to technical, scientific Medicine as such. In the last analysis there is as much difference between Christians and non-Christians practising routine, technical Medicine as there is between their servicing a car and tuning a carburettor. Both forms of duty can be fatal if not done with skill and thoroughness. But there is a difference — an immense difference — between the outlook of a Christian man and a non-Christian. It is so obvious that we tend to overlook it. The Christian is (or should be) from beginning to end Christ's man — learning His will, seeking to please Him, obeying His commands and wholly at His disposal. Could anything change a man more than such a new total allegiance? Whilst this will not change his technical Medicine or scientific ability, it will change his chief hopes and aspirations, his attitudes and way of life. *We are not doctors who happen to be Christians, but Christians who happen to be doctors.* . . . Certainly a Christian doctor is different from a non-Christian doctor, because a Christian is different from a non-Christian.'

'Where differences will begin to show will be in individual interpretations of life and the world, their outside interests and use of leisure, and their more intimate advice on matters outside Medicine. In other words, the difference is not in Medicine but in the men themselves who are practising it. It appears in the doctor's view of the nature of man, his explanation of the great contradiction between the good which man desires and the evil which he so constantly meets and practises. It shows itself in attitudes to disease, death and man's ultimate destiny; and in differences of motivation for service and the goals attempted. The divergence lies in their intimate personal outlooks as distinct from their professional service, competence and patient care.'

THE CRUX

The basic outlook of thousands of Christian doctors and nurses down the centuries was put in striking form by John M. Gray in his final report to the International Grenfell Association after 23 years as physician on the Newfoundland and Labrador coasts. He quoted from William Park's *Every Man his own Doctor* (subtitled *The Poor Planter's Physician* — published from his own printing press in Williamsburg in 1734, price one shilling). Park wrote: 'The most acceptable service we render to God is beneficence to man. There are three ways of benefiting our fellow creatures. We may be useful to their souls, by good instruction and good example. We may be helpful to their bodies by feeding the hungry, clothing the naked and prescribing useful remedies to the sick. We can aid them in their fortunes by encouragement of industry, by relieving the distressed, and doing all the kind offices we are able to our neighbours. These are the simple ways of improving the talents our Maker has entrusted us with; and we must expect hereafter to give an account how we have used them.'

In a similar vein Thomas Sydenham reminded those who take up Medicine 'that such skill and science as, by the blessing of Almighty God, he has allowed, are to be specially directed towards the good of his fellow-creatures: since it is a base thing for the great gifts of heaven to become the servants of avarice and ambition . . . He must remember that it is no mean or ignoble animal that he deals with . . . since for its sake God's only begotten Son became man, and thereby ennobled the nature he took upon Him.'

The willingness and persistence of a Christian practitioner to maintain such service throughout his professional life depends upon his having a rock-like conviction about one great fact. J. B. Lightfoot of Durham, the most revered and scholarly English bishop of the 19th century, sums it up in his *Biblical Essays on the Authenticity of St. John's Gospel:* 'I believe from my heart that the truth which this Gospel of John more especially enshrines — the truth that Jesus Christ is the very Word incarnate, the manifestation of the Father to mankind — is the one lesson which, duly apprehended, will do more than all our feeble efforts to purify and elevate human life here by imparting to it hope, and light and strength; the one study which alone can fitly prepare us for a joyful immortality hereafter.'

BIBLIOGRAPHY OF CHIEF SOURCES CONSULTED

1. GENERAL REFERENCE

Dictionary of National Biography, London, 1882 and series.
Kelly, E. C., Encyclopaedia of Medical Sources, Baltimore, 1948.
Kelly, H. A. Cyclopaedia of American Medical Biography, New York, 1928 (two vols).
Munk, W., Roll of Royal College of Physicians, London, 1878 and series.
Plarr, V. G., Lives of the Fellows of the Royal College of Surgeons of England, London, 1930 and series.
Schmidt, J. E., Medical Discoveries, Who and When, a Dictionary, Springfield, 1959.
Thornton, J. L., Mark, A. J. and Brooke, E. S., A Select Bibliography of Medical Biography, London, 1961.

2. GENERAL HISTORIES OF MEDICINE

Castiglioni, A., A History of Medicine, New York, 1947.
Garrison, F. H., Introduction to the History of Medicine, Philadelphia, 1929.
Guthrie, D., A History of Medicine, London, 1958.
Pollak, K. and Underwood, E. A., The Healers: The Doctor Then and Now, London, 1968.
Singer, C. and Underwood, E. A., A Short History of Medicine, Oxford, 1962.
Venzmer, G., Five Thousand Years of Medicine, London, 1972.

3. NATIONAL HISTORIES

Comrie, J. D., History of Scottish Medicine (two vols), London, 1932.
Fleetwood, J., History of Medicine in Ireland, Dublin, 1951.
Friedenwald, H., The Jews in Medicine, Baltimore, 1944.

Jaramillo-Arango, J., The British Contribution to Medicine, Edinburgh 1953.

Packard, F. R., History of Medicine in the United States, New York (two vols), 1931.

Poynter, F. N. L., The Evolution of Medical Practice in Britain, London, 1961.

Poynter, F. N. L., The Evolution of the Hospital in Britain, London, 1964.

Poynter, F. N. L., The Evolution of Medical Education in Britain, London 1966.

4. HISTORIES OF INSTITUTIONS

Cameron, H. C., Mr Guy's Hospital, London, 1954.

Clarke, G., History of the Royal College of Physicians, Oxford, 1964.

Clark Kennedy, A. E., The London Hospital, London 1962.

Clay, R. M., The Mediaeval Hospitals of England, London, 1909.

Dainton, C., The Story of England's Hospitals, London, 1961.

Davidson, M., Medicine in Oxford, Oxford, 1953.

Dewhurst, K., Oxford Medicine, Oxford, 1970.

Duncan, A., Memorials of the Faculty of Medicine and Surgery of Glasgow, Glasgow, 1896.

Harley, H., The Royal Society: Its Origin and Founders, London 1960.

Humble, J. G. and Hansell, P., Westminster Hospital, 1716-1966, London, 1966.

Hunt, T., History of the Medical Society of London, London, 1973.

Ives, A. J. L., British Hospitals, London, 1948.

Power, D'Arcy, British Medical Societies, London, 1939.

Rook, A., Cambridge and Its Contribution to Medicine, London, 1971.

Williams, W. H., America's First Hospital, Philadelphia, 1976.

5. SECTIONAL HISTORIES

Bishop, W. J., The Early History of Surgery, London, 1960.

Carr-Saunders, A. M. and Wilson, P. A., The Professions, London, 1964.

Chesterman, C. C., In the Service of Suffering (Medical Missions), London, 1940.

Dock, L. L. and Stewart, I., A Short History of Nursing, New York, 1920.

Dodd, E., The Gift of the Healer (Medical Missions), New York, 1920.

Fulton, J., Selected Readings in Physiology, Springfield, 1930.

Gordon, B. L., Medicine through Antiquity, Philadelphia, 1949.

Gordon, B. L., Mediaeval and Renaissance Medicine, London, 1960.

Heasman, K., The Evangelicals in Action, London, 1962.

Heller, R., Priest-Doctors: a rural health service *Medical History 20,* 361, London, 1976.

Hooykaas, R., Religion and the Rise of Science, Edinburgh, 1972.

Hunter, R. and Macalpine, J., Three Hundred Years of British Psychiatry, Oxford, 1963.

Leigh, D., Historical Development of British Psychiatry, Oxford, 1961.

Pavey, A. E., The Story of the Growth of Nursing, London, 1938.

Rosenberg, C., Healing and History, New York, 1979.

Scott, H. H., History of Tropical Medicine, London (two vols), 1939.

Sigerist, H. E., On the Sociology of Medicine, New York, 1960.

Still, F. S., The History of Paediatrics, London, 1931.

Wain, H., History of Preventive Medicine, Springfield, 1970.

Watson, G., Theriac and Mithridatium, London, 1966.

Webster, C., The Great Instauration, London, 1975.

Williams, G., The Age of Miracles, London, 1981.

6 COLLECTIONS OF SHORT BIOGRAPHIES

Bailey, H. and Bishop, W. J., Notable Names in Medicine and Surgery, London, 1959.

Macmichael, W., Lives of British Physicians, London, 1830.

Power, D'Arcy, British Masters of Medicine, London, 1936.

Sigerist, H. E., Great Doctors: A Biographical History of Medicine, London, 1933.

7 BIOGRAPHIES

Abraham, J. J., Lettsom: His Life and Times, London, 1933.

Barlow, A., Sir Thomas Barlow, London, 1965.

Beall, O. T. and Shryock, R. H., Cotton Mather, Baltimore, 1954.

Clark, R. A. and Elkington, J. R., The Quaker Heritage in Medicine, London 1978.

Cushing, H., The Life of Sir William Osler, Oxford, 1940.

Deacon, M., Philip Doddridge of Northampton, Northampton, 1980.

Dewhurst, K., Thomas Sydenham, London, 1966.

Fisk, D., Jenner of Berkeley, London, 1959.

Fox, H., Dr John Fothergill and His Friends, London, 1919.

Godlee, R. J., Lord Lister, London, 1917.

Guy, W. A., John Howard's Winter Journey, London, 1882.

Hamly, W. B., Ambroise Paré, St. Louis, 1967.

Hector, Winifred, The Work of Mrs Bedford Fenwick, London, 1973.

Keynes, G., Ambroise Paré, London, 1951.

Keynes, G., William Harvey, Oxford, 1966.

Keynes, G., Sir Thomas Browne: Selected Writings, London, 1962.

Lennox-Kerr, J., Wilfred Grenfell, London, 1959.

Lindeboom, G. A., Hermann Boerhaave, London, 1968.

More, L. T., Life and Works of Robert Boyle, London, 1944.

Paget, S., Memoirs and Letters of James Paget, London, 1901.

Vallery-Radot, R., The Life of Pasteur, London, 1901.

Wagner, G., Barnardo, London, 1979.

Williams, A. E., Barnardo of Stepney, London, 1946.

Wilson, R. M., The Beloved Physician (James Mackenzie), London, 1926.

INDEX OF PERSONAL NAMES

INDEX OF SUBJECTS AND PLACES